The Evolution and Legacy of the Engel and Romano Work in Biopsychosocial Medicine

The Evolution and Legacy of the Engel and Romano Work in Biopsychosocial Medicine

Diane S. Morse,
Katherine R. Johnson,
and Jules Cohen

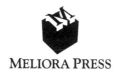

MELIORA PRESS
An imprint of the University of Rochester Press

First published 2013

Meliora Press is an imprint of the
University of Rochester Press
668 Mt. Hope Avenue, Rochester, NY 14620, USA
www.urpress.com
and Boydell & Brewer Limited
PO Box 9, Woodbridge, Suffolk IP12 3DF, UK
www.boydellandbrewer.com

ISBN-13: 978-1-58046-470-3

Library of Congress Cataloging-in-Publication Data

Morse, Diane S., author.
    The evolution and legacy of the Engel and Romano work in biopsychoso-
cial medicine / Diane S. Morse, Katherine R. Johnson, and Jules Cohen.
        p. ; cm.
    Includes bibliographical references and index.
    ISBN 978-1-58046-470-3 (hbk. : alk. paper)
    I. Johnson, Katherine R., author. II. Cohen, Jules, 1931– author. III. Title.
    [DNLM: 1. Engel, George L. (George Libman), 1913–1999.
2. Romano, John, 1908–1994. 3. University of Rochester. School of
Medicine and Dentistry. 4. Psychosomatic Medicine—education.
5. Curriculum. 6. Education, Medical—history. 7. History, 20th Century.
8. Models, Psychological. 9. Psychiatry—Biography. 10. Social
Medicine—education. WM 18]
    RC464.A1
    616.890092'2—dc23   2013019609

This publication is printed on acid-free paper.
Printed in the United States of America.

*To the memory of George Engel and John Romano,
in recognition of their vision and powerful
inspiration as teachers and mentors.*

Contents

Acknowledgments

The authors are greatly indebted to the physicians, researchers, and educators at Rochester and elsewhere who shared with us their insights and knowledge about George Engel, John Romano, Rochester's liaison unit and fellowship, and biopsychosocial medicine teaching and research at Rochester and beyond: Robert Ader, Eric Caine, Thomas Campbell, Douglas Drossman, Ronald Epstein, Shimon Glick, Laurence Guttmacher, David Lambert, Mack Lipkin, Kathryn Markakis, Susan McDaniel, Jan Moynihan, Dennis Novack, Timothy Quill, Dorith Shaham, and Geoffrey Williams.

We are very grateful to Christopher Hoolihan, history of medicine librarian and archivist at the Edward G. Miner Library at the University of Rochester Medical Center; Theodore Brown, professor of history, public health sciences, and medical humanities at Rochester; Stephanie Brown Clark, director of Rochester's Division of Medical Humanities and Bioethics; Amy Gregory, Jules Cohen's secretary; Margaret Downen in the Office of Medical Education; and Maria Milella of the Palliative Care Program.

I

Roots of Rochester's Program in Biopsychosocial Medicine

Two texts serve as the background for this monograph: Professor Theodore Brown's detailed paper, "The Historical and Conceptual Foundations of the Rochester Biopsychosocial Model," and the historical biography by Jules Cohen and Stephanie Brown Clark, *John Romano and George Engel: Their Lives and Work.*[1]

As both sources reveal, the roots of Rochester's biopsychosocial (BPS) model go back to about 1940, when John Romano and George Engel first came together in Boston. Romano was a young faculty member trained in psychiatry at Yale and Colorado, appointed to work at Harvard's Peter Bent Brigham Hospital (PBBH) by Soma Weiss, chair of the Department of Medicine. Weiss was a very broadly oriented clinical teacher and physician-scientist who was highly supportive of Romano's research into the psychological and behavioral aspects of disease. Romano wrote, "I saw Soma Weiss as a superb teacher, clinician and humanist . . . giving me insight into a broad humanistic approach to a sick person, and in being a doctor at the bedside. . . . I feel that I have been made a better doctor and a better person for having known and worked with Soma Weiss."[2]

In contrast to Romano, whose upbringing was modest, Engel grew up in the well-to-do Upper East Side of New York City in the home of his distinguished uncle, internist and research scientist Emmanuel Libman. Influenced by his uncle's scientific orientation as well as by his own medical school experience at Johns Hopkins, Engel developed a strong biomedical research orientation from early in his youth. After his internal medicine residency at New York's Mt. Sinai Hospital, he came to Boston to serve as a research fellow with Weiss, whose distinguished contributions to medicine and skills as a mentor Engel had come to appreciate when he had the opportunity to do research with Weiss during a medical school summer.

Weiss appreciated both Romano's breadth and his belief that it was important for physicians to be "broadly civilized." He urged Engel to accompany Romano on rounds and see whether Romano's wisdom and integrative approach could expand Engel's orientation and perhaps result in a productive collaboration.

Initially resistant but urged on by Weiss, Engel agreed. He observed Romano at rounds, conducting patient interviews that focused on the patient's *personal* story rather than on merely the biology of the disease process. The patient's symptoms in his or her own words—and the life circumstances that may have influenced the onset and course of illness—informed Romano's careful clinical evaluation. Engel was greatly impressed by both Romano and the central power of the in-depth interview in eliciting psychosocial information. He later commented: "I saw the attending, John Romano, a young psychiatrist, pull up a chair, and sit down with the patient and, in effect, invite him to tell his own story before the assembled group. . . . The daring of Weiss's thinking and the drama of Romano's 'pulling up a chair' and listening to the patient, as he was accustomed to do on psychiatric rounds, changed my life forever. My entire career since can be traced to that happy concordance of vision and action."[3] Romano and Engel began working together, initially on delirium. Romano became impressed with Engel, and, when appointed chair of psychiatry at the University of Cincinnati, he invited Engel to join him there.

In Cincinnati, Engel finally came to acknowledge the relevance of psychological matters in illness and clinical care. There, he and Romano continued their work on delirium. Working with internists Eugene Ferris and Chair of Medicine Marion Blankenhorn, they also studied the role of psychological factors in the precipitation of decompression symptoms ("the bends") in subjects recovering from low-pressure exposure in a decompression chamber. This work not only furthered their research collaborations but also brought them together in efforts to build attention to psychological factors in health and illness into the school's teaching programs. While Ferris and some senior faculty in psychiatry (for example, Maurice Levine and Milton Rosenbaum) shared these interests, many in the school did not and were resistant. Therefore, when George Whipple, dean of the medical school at the University of Rochester, invited Romano to become founding chair of Rochester's Department of Psychiatry—and indicated that Rochester would welcome Romano's and Engel's efforts to teach the psychosocial dimension of patient care—Romano enthusiastically accepted the offer and invited Engel to join him. When (in contrast to Blankenhorn) William McCann, Rochester's chair of medicine, expressed receptiveness to their ideas, Romano and Engel became even more enthusiastic about coming to Rochester.

II

Foundations of Rochester's Biopsychosocial Curriculum

Soon after he arrived in Rochester in 1946, Romano created and taught the first-year course in psychosocial medicine (PSM), Fundamental Concepts of Human Behavior. The course dealt with the influence of genetic, physiological, psychological, and social forces on the development of personality, as well as the interplay between adaptive forces and significant psychological influences on health maintenance and illness. The negative effects of psychological stress on one's sense of well-being had long been appreciated. But the idea that family, financial, work-related, and other personal stressors could precipitate illness was a new concept Romano introduced to students in this course.

During the same time, Engel designed and directed the second-year course in psychosocial medicine, Medical Psychology and Psychopathology, and he was strongly supported by Romano in this undertaking. Engel's goal was to expose students to an array of clinical problems and to demonstrate, through in-depth interviews of patients, the psychological, behavioral, and social—as well as biomedical—factors and forces affecting patients' health and the onset and course of illness.[1] He gave particular attention to the role of physicians in modifying those factors.[2] His work in this course, which was renamed Psychosocial Medicine II (PSM II), and the concepts he taught were later expressed in his formulation of the BPS model.[3]

In addition to the impact of introducing these pioneering concepts in the first- and second-year courses, Romano and Engel had a broader influence on institutional culture through their teaching

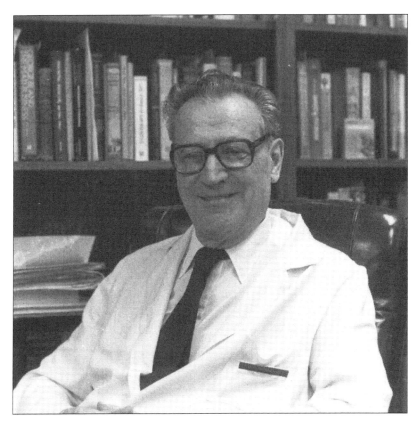

Figure 1. John Romano, 1974

on internal medicine and other *clinical* services, through Engel's establishment of the Medical-Psychiatric Liaison Unit and Fellowship, and in the work of psychosocially oriented liaison faculty and fellows (see chapter 4).[4] Engel's influence spread further through the General Clerkship, an innovative program for third-year medical students that he and Professor of Medicine William Morgan created. This course emphasized teaching the basic clinical skills of history taking and physical examination, the crucial role of effective physician-patient communication in an in-depth, patient-centered interview, and the importance of these skills in gaining a full understanding of the biological and psychosocial factors affecting patients' health.[5]

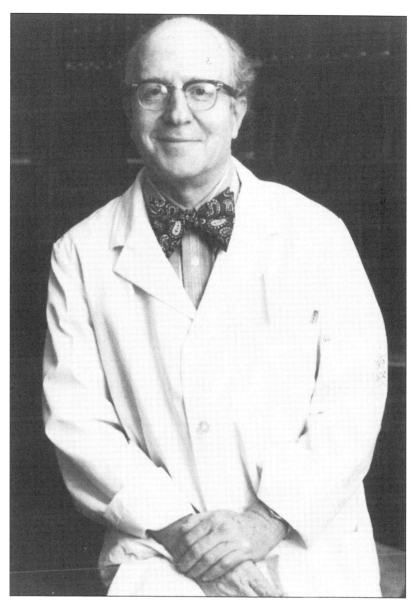

Figure 2. George Engel, 1975

When Engel stepped down as director of PSM II in the early 1980s, he hoped to be succeeded by an internist who was also interested in having an impact on the way students conducted medical histories. Romano had retired as chair of psychiatry, however, and the new departmental leadership appointed psychiatrists to run the course. Engel's immediate successor, David Rosen, maintained the course's traditional structure and BPS orientation.[6] During the same era, Rosen was also involved in designing and teaching a new interdisciplinary course, Introduction to Human Health and Illness, a program of whole case conferences with a strong BPS focus.[7] This course was created as part of the medical school's curriculum restructuring in the early 1980s led by Jules Cohen, a Romano-Engel disciple appointed senior associate dean for medical education in 1982. When Rosen left Rochester in the late 1980s, he was succeeded by Otto Thaler, a psychoanalytically oriented psychiatrist who had trained under Romano and been highly regarded by students as director of PSM I. The next director, Laurence Guttmacher, also a psychiatrist, spearheaded an interdisciplinary approach and recruited generalist and primary care faculty with BPS interests to teach small-group sessions and thus help maintain some of the course's integrative BPS orientation.[8] But the course had changed. Engel's distinctive mode of interviewing had led students, regardless of the specialty they intended to pursue, to see the patient as a whole, and his strong leadership had prevented the BPS approach from being marginalized to the specialty of psychiatry. Even though his successors had been somewhat successful in their efforts to replicate the structure and orientation of the course, they had trained as psychiatrists, and—most important—they were not Engel.

Curriculum Change in the Late 1990s

In 1997 Edward Hundert replaced Jules Cohen as senior associate dean for medical education and shepherded another major revision of the curriculum. Although a new "double-helix" curriculum was structured to be more interdisciplinary and integrative, it arguably resulted in a diminution of BPS teaching. Hundert and other curriculum planners thought both PSM I and PSM II could be eliminated and that a BPS orientation could be included adequately in weekly "integration conferences."[9] Although some biopsychosocially oriented faculty opposed this move and saw it as a threat to BPS teaching, others favored the integration conferences, arguing that students would not then see BPS medicine as separate from "regular" medicine.[10] After some negotiation, the dedicated year-long psychosocial medicine courses for first- and second-year students were eliminated.

Planners also hoped three other courses would help teach BPS medicine concepts. They created two new programs—Introduction to Clinical Medicine for first-year students and Mind, Brain, and Behavior in the second year—and expanded and modified the Ambulatory Care Experience, a practice-based teaching program for preclinical students that had begun in the late 1980s.

In teaching programs for third- and fourth-year students, a major change in BPS education came with the elimination of the General Clerkship. The fairly heavy involvement of liaison faculty in that program thus ended, further diminishing biopsychosocially oriented teaching. Furthermore, without Engel's involvement, there was no influential champion of the BPS approach in the clinical years. Some faculty members believe this also resulted in an erosion of interviewing and physical diagnosis instruction in the Rochester curriculum.[11]

III

Current Biopsychosocial Medicine
Teaching at Rochester

First- and Second-Year Programs

Introduction to Clinical Medicine is taught from August to December of the first year. Created by Nancy S. Clark in 1999, the course is now directed by Eric Richard. Timothy Quill, who trained under Engel as a liaison fellow, is a key faculty member.[1] Based on experiences with inpatients and standardized patients, students develop skills in the patient-centered interview, such as learning the patient's perspective, discerning the patient's agenda, and showing empathy when obtaining a medical history. Attitudinal goals of the course include development of professionalism, self-awareness, humanism, compassion, honesty, and integrity—all of which are central values in the BPS approach.[2]

The Primary Care Clerkship (PCC) is the cornerstone of clinical instruction in the first two years. Originally called the Ambulatory Clerkship Experience, its first course director, appointed in 1999, was Kathryn Markakis—an internist who had trained as a liaison fellow under Timothy Quill, Anthony Suchman, and Professor Emeritus Engel. Eventually, it was restructured and renamed PCC. In 2011 family medicine's Anne Nofziger became course director, with Markakis staying on as assistant course director.[3]

PCC places students with primary care physicians from March of the first year to the end of the second year. The didactic portion of the program is largely topic-driven and covers the basics of prevention, acute care, and chronic disease management for the most common conditions seen in primary care practices. Workshop sessions reinforce interviewing and physical exam skills learned earlier in the first year and provide practice in examining and evaluating patients in standardized, small-group settings, which include video recording and playback capabilities in each teaching room. In addition, weekly integration conferences bring a significant BPS focus to the evaluation of a variety of actual patients.[4]

The second-year portion of PCC includes Master Clinician Rounds, taught by community internists, family physicians, and full-time clinical faculty—some of whom completed medical school, biopsychosocially oriented residencies, or a liaison fellowship at Rochester (e.g., Michael Krasner, Diane Morse, and Anthony Suchman).[5] Students are observed as they interview inpatients, outpatients, or standardized patients; and they present a case from their continuity outpatient experiences. Explicit attention is paid to clinical reasoning and evidence-based medicine, emphasizing Engel and Romano's approach to interviewing, regardless of the clinical problem.

A question worthy of discussion is whether biopsychosocially oriented interviewing can really be taught with standardized patients, in contrast to the Romano-Engel interviews of genuine patients. Engel and Romano might have argued that interviewing a so-called standardized patient cannot uncover the subtle, patient-specific psychosocial issues of a real patient. Some who knew both men felt they would have accepted only actual patients for teaching medical students. Others, however, believe they would have embraced the unique teaching and research opportunities afforded by the use of knowledgeable, professional standardized patients who can provide feedback and help students and others practice interviewing.[6] In Rochester's program, standardized patients have been trained in traditional clinical as well as BPS skills. In addition, student sessions with standardized patients use active, self-directed learning formats, which adult learning theories suggest are more effective.[7] Further, research supports the use of standardized patients in teaching, including in comparisons with experiences using actual patients.[8]

Mind, Brain, and Behavior is a nine-week course in the second year initially conceived as a third new program to help substitute for the psychosocial medicine courses and integrate with study of the neural sciences. Neurologist Ralph Jozefowicz, the very popular and effective course director of the former neural sciences course, was appointed to design and direct Mind, Brain, and Behavior—working with Jeffrey Lyness, a geropsychiatrist and Rochester medical school graduate.[9] The program is a multidisciplinary introduction to the human nervous system, integrating basic science and clinical disciplines. Both basic science and clinical faculty teach in lectures, laboratories, and problem-based learning cases; and weekly integration conferences focus on neurological and psychiatric disorders. The course aims to familiarize students with the complex interplay of biological, psychological, and social factors in the genesis and management of psychiatric disorders and emphasizes the importance of excellence in history and physical examination.

Third- and Fourth-Year Student Experiences

Students in third- and fourth-year clerkships and externships in internal medicine, pediatrics, and family medicine learn integrative skills through exposure to preceptors and residents familiar with the BPS model from their own training at Rochester. According to Valerie Lang, director of the internal medicine clerkship, a significant number of current clerkship faculty had such exposure.[10] In addition, clinical students have contact with a number of preceptors who view stress reduction and self-awareness as important components of patient care.[11] This approach resonates with Engel's psychoanalytic perspective in medical interviewing and addressing countertransference in the patient encounter.[12]

Teaching Programs in Medical Humanities, Bioethics, Health Law, and Palliative Care

These programs give expression first to Romano's belief that the broadly civilized physician is better equipped to provide humane care to patients. These educational efforts relate closely to Romano's many writings on ethics, scientific integrity, the physician's social responsibilities, and applications of the humanities to medical education.[13] Such programs also complement other BPS initiatives at Rochester and help physicians-in-training enhance their communication skills, providing a direct linkage to Engel's work.

A program in the medical humanities began in the late 1970s with a series of classes for first-year students taught by founding director Kathryn Montgomery, a newly appointed faculty member with an interest in literature related to medicine.[14] The program was soon expanded to include offerings on the history of medicine and philosophy as related to medicine, and faculty members from the Departments of History and Philosophy in the College of Arts and Sciences were recruited to teach some of these classes. The program was further enriched in the early 1980s by the appointment of Jane Greenlaw, an attorney with a background in nursing, who assumed leadership responsibility for programs in her fields of expertise in medical ethics and health law.[15] When Greenlaw retired in 2012, Marjorie Hodges Shaw, an attorney who also holds a PhD from Rochester's Warner School of Education, was appointed to direct the programs in bioethics and law.[16]

With the 1998 appointment of Stephanie Brown Clark, an MD/PhD with expertise in medical history and literature in medicine, the programs expanded to include new electives in medicine-related literature, including drama.[17] Brown Clark now oversees Rochester's

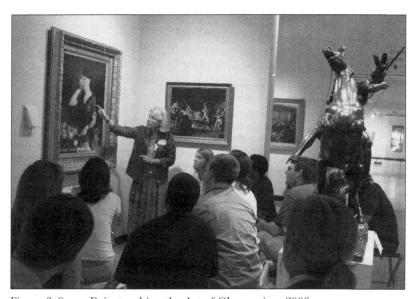

Figure 3. Susan Daiss teaching the Art of Observation, 2006

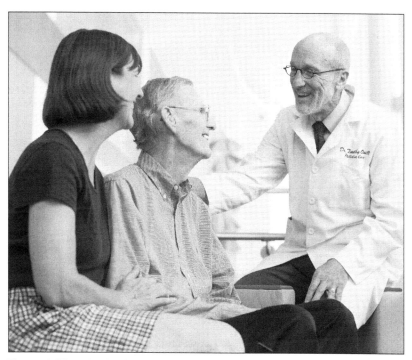

Figure 4. Timothy Quill with a palliative care patient, 2012

medical humanities programs, which address key issues in medicine by applying methodologies and materials from various disciplines—including history, visual arts, philosophy, music, and film, as well as studies in gender, religion, culture, and disabilities. For example, in the Reader's Theatre Group, interested students, residents, and faculty take roles in or observe plays adapted from authors such as Chekov, featuring ethical and professional issues in medical care. In addition, in cooperation with Susan Daiss, director of education at the University's Memorial Art Gallery, the division offers the Art of Observation, an innovative program designed to enhance students' observational skills through the study of great works of art.

The Palliative Care Program, which began in 2001 under Timothy Quill's leadership, has become a vital component of the school's teaching programs. It includes a highly respected consultative clinical service with fellows, nurse practitioners, and physicians from internal medicine, family medicine, geriatrics, neurology, pediatrics, and oncology. This staff offers a rich array of educational programs to medical students and residents in internal medicine and medicine-pediatrics, as well as fellows in a palliative care program certified by the Accreditation Council for Graduate Medical Education. Staff members also conduct an active research program and have written leading-edge scholarly papers on palliative and end-of-life care.[18]

All of the interdisciplinary programs in the medical humanities, bioethics, health law, and palliative care focus on families as well as individual patients. In addition to centrally involved faculty (Brown Clark, Greenlaw, Shaw, and Quill), a substantial number of other interested faculty members have held secondary appointments in these areas, making valued and manifold contributions to the BPS tradition.

Family Medicine's Expanded Role in Biopsychosocial Teaching

Rochester's Department of Family Medicine plays a central role in biopsychosocially oriented medical student education, in collaboration with the Departments of Internal Medicine and Pediatrics. These collaborations grew out of a changing institutional culture at Rochester, reflecting a national trend over the last thirty or forty years of greater receptivity to the role of family medicine in medical education. Family medicine as a discipline has an inherently BPS orientation in its integration of societal as well as individual and family emotional contexts into the care of families, an orientation John Romano had long advocated.[19] Family medicine departments across the country articulate BPS values in their early clinical teaching programs. In addition, they incorporate biopsychosocially oriented approaches into their later clerkships, as well as their clinical practice and research activities.

As he entered his emeritus years, Engel hoped greater involvement of family medicine would help keep the medical school biopsychosocially oriented. His own interest in family-systems approaches was growing and fit well with his psychoanalytic approach to understanding both his own family and that of Monica, an infant with a gastric fistula who was the subject of decades-long studies by

Engel and his colleague, Franz Reichsman (see chapter 4). Engel also began to look at the tapes from the Monica studies from the perspective of family effects.[20] In the 1980s he arranged meetings to discuss weaving family medicine approaches and BPS teaching into the school's overall educational programs.[21] Romano also had interests in family issues, as reflected in his longitudinal study of schizophrenic patients and their families.[22]

The late-in-life change in Engel's orientation to family-systems approaches is revealed in a Diane Morse interview with him published in 1996 in the journal *Families, Systems, & Health* and in an article he authored in the same issue.[23] Engel observed that what was formerly medicine-psychiatry had become medicine, psychiatry, and family medicine, with a greater orientation toward community health issues.[24] This philosophical change was important to the expansion of Rochester's educational programs in community-based care in the 1980s—and to the *early* ambulatory care clinical experiences for all medical students introduced in the double-helix curriculum in the late 1990s.

IV

Medical-Psychiatric Liaison Unit and Fellowship

In 1946, soon after he and John Romano arrived in Rochester, George Engel developed the Medical-Psychiatric Liaison Unit and Fellowship. He had strong support for this undertaking from Romano and William McCann, chair of the Department of Medicine. For over thirty years, the unit and fellowship played vital roles in biopsychosocially oriented teaching, clinical care, and research, attracting top-quality physicians—mostly internists—to serve as faculty and fellows.

The teaching and research contributions of senior faculty members of the Medical-Psychiatric Liaison Unit (e.g., William Greene, Arthur Schmale, Sanford Meyerowitz, Franz Reichsman, and others) were centrally important in developing and sustaining the institutional BPS culture. Most important was their impact on the students, residents, and fellows they taught.

Building on the formative influence of John Romano and George Engel, liaison faculty focused on the critical importance, in both teaching and research, of high-quality patient-centered interviews in understanding the onset and course of illness. In particular, they came to appreciate the important pathophysiological role of personal loss, such as clinical depression, death of a family member or close friend, having to leave a longtime home, or major financial loss—including dissolution of a business. They came to understand that such life stressors, especially in combination, were capable of setting the conditions for the onset of a major illness—for example, a significant cardiovascular event (such as an acute myocardial infarction, serious arrhythmia, or stroke), gastrointestinal ulcer, colitis,

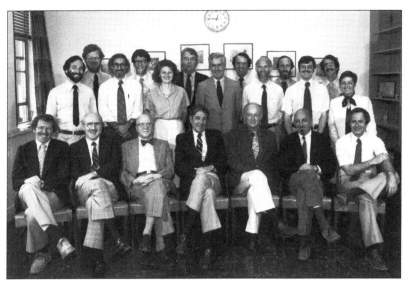

Figure 5. Medical-Psychiatric Liaison Unit, 1980–81

major infection, autoimmune disorder (such as rheumatoid arthritis), or malignancy. Faculty members sought out patients with these disorders for study and carefully explored the psychobiologic relationships between "life loss" and the onset or progression of illness.

William Greene, for example, working with members of the Hematology Unit faculty, explored these relationships in patients with lymphoma and leukemia.[1] In addition, working with Cardiology Unit faculty, he researched and developed an understanding of stressful life events that seemed to play a role in precipitating sudden cardiac death or myocardial infarction.[2] An extraordinary turn of events gave very personal expression to Greene's theories when he was scheduled to present the results of his work at a Cardiology Unit research studies meeting early one evening. When no one showed up promptly, Greene became *very* agitated, thinking that no one in cardiology was interested in hearing about his research. He went out into the hallway next to the conference room to see where everyone was and then collapsed. Fortuitously, a senior medical resident saw him, called a "code," and began resuscitation efforts. Within minutes, many of the cardiology faculty arrived, and ventricular fibrillation was documented. After several anxious moments, Greene was successfully defibrillated and admitted to the Coronary Care Unit, where he recovered. He lived for many symptom-free years following this event and ultimately succumbed to complications of cerebral vascular disease.

Arthur Schmale explored the relationships between life loss and the clinical appearance and progression of various illnesses, including malignancies. As part of an early study of these interactions, he reviewed the extensive literature documenting the relationship between depression and the onset of illness.[3] When his work later focused on the importance of psychological factors in the onset of various malignancies, he and George Engel formulated a psychoanalytic basis for the observed relationships between life loss, depression, hopelessness, and illness onset and progression.[4]

Sanford Meyerowitz, working with faculty members in rheumatology, studied the role of psychological factors in the rheumatic disorders.[5] His general expertise in education led to his appointment as the first associate dean for medical education at Rochester and his influential role in developing the Rochester Plan in the early 1970s. The Rochester Plan (Early Selection Program), supported by the Commonwealth Fund, was an innovative program that fostered linkages between the medical school and the university as a whole and responded to Commonwealth's urging to lessen "the barriers between the basic sciences in the medical schools and the natural and behavioral sciences in the parent universities."[6] In the Rochester Plan, which aimed to integrate baccalaureate and medical education experiences, selected undergraduates created their own eight-year programs, which wove medical school courses into their last two baccalaureate years and baccalaureate courses into their first two years of medical school. Students were encouraged to craft distinctive, highly enriched, and innovative programs of study. Those accepted into the Rochester Plan had early assurance of admission to the medical school. The aim was to graduate a core of physicians with scholarly and personal breadth and enable students to avoid redundancies in their scientific preparation for medicine while enriching and broadening their educational experiences during both the baccalaureate and medical school years. Much of the program's creative design flowed from Meyerowitz's thinking. In addition, after he retired as chair of psychiatry, John

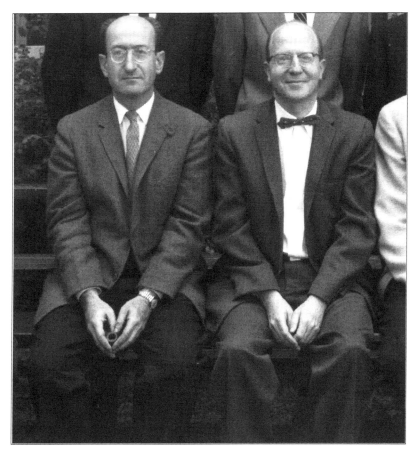

Figure 6. Franz Reichsman and George Engel, 1963

Romano became very involved in the Rochester Plan, advising students and ensuring that the program's goals were being met.

The psychoanalytic roots of some of the work by liaison faculty members can be found in Engel and Franz Reichsman's earlier long-term studies of gastric secretion in Monica and other infants with gastric fistulae. They conducted research into the physiological, psychological, and behavioral relationships between gastric secretion and psychological development and examined spontaneous and histamine-induced gastric secretion in depression, withdrawal states, coma, sleep, and when the subjects were highly engaged with the experimenter.[7] Reichsman was also a wise and favorite mentor of medical students and a highly effective teacher at the bedside, and it was a considerable loss to Rochester when he left to become head of the medical-psychiatric program at the Downstate Medical School in Brooklyn.

The congeniality of Engel and Reichsman's relationship is revealed in a story that also shows Engel's occasional preoccupation with his personal accomplishments. At a dinner with friends, where he was holding forth in characteristic fashion about his work, all the places he had been invited to speak, and the many awards he had received (while people around the table were rolling their eyes), Reichsman brought things to a hilarious standstill by joking, "Well, George, did you know that Freud was at my bar mitzvah?" Everyone, including Engel, was convulsed with laughter.

Liaison faculty and fellows were a constant presence on the medical service of the medical school's main teaching hospital, Strong Memorial Hospital. They saw almost all admitted patients with medical students and residents, conducted weekly liaison teaching rounds for third-year medical students, and provided suggestions regarding patient care—especially when psychological factors were important in patients' clinical presentations. By the mid-1970s, however, the program's success was in some ways its undoing. First, although fellows included well-trained internists, family physicians, and gynecologists, medical residents came to view them as psychiatrists, and their suggestions were greeted skeptically or simply dismissed. Second, their constant presence was felt to be excessive and intrusive, interfering with residents' independence and responsibilities.[8] In addition, new leadership in the Department of Medicine was less supportive of the BPS approach and responded to the residents' concerns by sharply curtailing liaison activities. Engel tried to reverse this, but he succeeded only in part. Romano had retired as chair of psychiatry, and his influence—though still substantial—could not be brought to bear on the conflict.

As a result of these restrictions to fellows' responsibilities, the program became a more traditional consultation-liaison fellowship. The clinical activities of fellows shifted from teaching students and residents to providing consultative services on the floors of the hospital for patients in whom psychological factors played an important role; therefore, fellows had to call on faculty psychiatrists to support their consultative efforts. As a result, the overall influence of Engel and other liaison faculty diminished. Still, they continued to play an important role, and the fellows appreciated their influence in bringing BPS thinking into both their approaches to patients and their scholarship.[9] Ultimately, the central objective of the fellowship—to prepare leaders in BPS education, clinical care, and research—was achieved, as exemplified by the accomplishments of Rolf Adler, Douglas Drossman, Ronald Epstein, Mack Lipkin, Dennis Novack, Timothy Quill, and others.[10]

Engel's approach to teaching fellows changed somewhat during these years. He became more personally engaged with them and more willing to serve as a mentor.[11] He invited them to his home for cookies and tea, reviewed and discussed the Monica tapes with them, and proudly showed them his wife's paintings. In end-of-year ceremonies, at which he expressed "fatherly" feelings toward the fellows, Engel presented them with personalized, signed copies of his well-known doodles, to which he was deeply attached.[12]

Fellows were also involved in the unit's research. Although Engel was a career NIH investigator, the research standards of the 1950s–70s were not those of the modern era. Drossman notes that Engel's research was very observational; he would gather information, look at commonalities, and try to explain them.[13] Engel's research mentoring, like his clinical supervision, was "loose." He was responsive but provided little guidance. When Novack had to shorten an article accepted by the *Journal of the American Medical Association*, Engel initially joked that every third paragraph could simply be deleted, but then he was quite helpful.[14]

Over time, liaison faculty and fellows faced challenges as research moved from clinically oriented observational studies and case reports to the type of basic science research done by Robert Ader and his colleagues, which demonstrated a link between psychological influences and immune function (see chapter 6).

Changes in the Leadership and Structure of the Medical-Psychiatric Liaison Unit and Fellowship

When Engel stepped down as head of the Medical-Psychiatric Liaison Unit in 1979, Arthur Schmale became acting head. A permanent replacement for Engel, however, was in question. Many believed Mack Lipkin had the vision and ability to continue the unit's influence in teaching and research and thus the potential to succeed him.[15] But Lipkin's relative youth and conflicts between these two strong personalities prevented that succession. There were financial, educational, clinical, and research issues rooted in differing philosophies, high expectations, and inevitable disappointments on both sides.[16] If Lipkin had continued at Rochester, Engel might well have wanted to oversee him, which would have perpetuated the conflict. As a result, Lipkin left in 1980 to pursue other opportunities and has been highly successful in promoting the growth and dissemination of BPS medicine.[17] David Rosen was also considered as a possible successor to Engel, but personality conflicts prevented this, too.[18] In addition, according to Thomas Campbell, a fellow in 1982–84, conflict had developed between the psychoanalytical orientation of liaison faculty and the behavioral orientation of the increasingly influential research faculty.[19] In 1982 the Medical-Psychiatric Liaison Unit was replaced by the Division of Behavioral and Psychosocial Medicine, and the basic-research-oriented Robert Ader was appointed director of the division and George L. Engel Professor of Psychosocial Medicine.[20] These changes in the unit's structure and leadership, as well as the departure of Rosen a few years later, left a less-than-welcoming atmosphere in the Department of Medicine for biopsychosocially oriented faculty and programs, as well as a gap in clinically oriented leadership to advocate for biopsychosocially inclined clinicians at the University of Rochester Medical Center (URMC).

Consequently, beginning in the early 1980s, the centers of gravity of the division's clinical and teaching efforts shifted to sites where those in family medicine and internal medicine with BPS orientations were based and where department chairs and senior leadership were supportive of the BPS approach: Genesee Hospital, at which Quill, Engel, Cecile Carson, and, later, Geoffrey Williams worked;[21] Highland Hospital, with Anthony Suchman, Howard Beckman, Richard Frankel, Ronald Epstein, Susan McDaniel, Thomas Campbell, Richard Botelho, and Kathryn Markakis;[22] and Rochester General Hospital, with Diane Morse. A strong relationship with the URMC remained, however, and funding initiatives for residency programs and fellowships in internal medicine and family medicine at Rochester in the 1980s and 1990s included some designated funds for biopsychosocially oriented faculty who were playing important teaching roles.[23] Since the early 1990s, after the leadership in the URMC's Department of Medicine changed and the priorities there became better matched, Quill and other like-minded faculty were attracted back to the medical center, where they have enhanced its BPS orientation. They have been more directly supported from financial sources there and through the NIH, even though in 2001 the URMC's Division of Behavioral and Psychosocial Medicine was dissolved as an academic unit.

The liaison fellowship underwent further changes. In the late 1980s and early 1990s, it was led by internist Quill at Genesee Hospital and internist Suchman and family physician Botelho, both at Highland Hospital. In these programs, fellows from the United States, Switzerland, China, and Norway studied together, giving internists training in family systems with McDaniel, Campbell, and others, while family physicians developed core medical interviewing skills with Suchman, Quill, Carson, Beckman, Frankel, and Engel. Although the fellowship is no longer offered, several Rochester faculty are former fellows, including Betty Rabinowitz, Diane Morse, Steven Novak, neurologist-ophthalmologist David N. Smith, Ronald Epstein, Geoffrey Williams, Kathryn Markakis, Anthony Suchman, and Timothy Quill.[24]

A recently created example of a biopsychosocially oriented training program is the fellowship in palliative medicine and end-of-life care at the URMC, led by Timothy Quill (described earlier). In his extraordinary dedication to teaching and practicing the in-depth interview, Quill is one of the most visible practitioners of Engel's legacy at Rochester. He made a four-part film of the in-depth interview as applied to end-of-life care, and the skills and spirit of the interview are derived from Engel's strategies. The palliative care fellowship is also an outgrowth of the liaison philosophy, in that faculty and learners are primary care physicians who focus on the special skills and importance of effective patient-physician communication that Engel and Romano believed should be practiced by physicians in all specialties, not just psychiatrists.

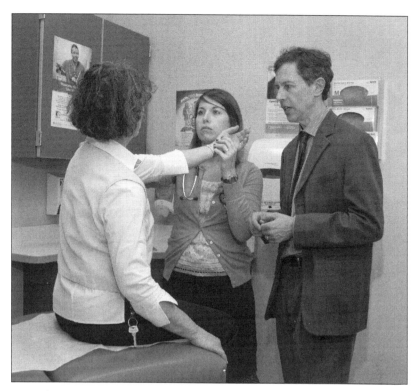

Figure 7. Ronald Epstein teaching a resident during a patient exam, 2012. Photograph by Vince Sullivan, University of Rochester Medical Center.

Another former fellow who has been a leader in BPS teaching and research at Rochester is Ronald Epstein. His prolific research has encompassed patient-centered care, the influence of patients on physicians' practice approaches, and physicians' self-awareness and mindfulness as they relate to difficult issues and at-risk and overlooked populations—for example, HIV-AIDS, somatization, and debilitating illness. He has designed groundbreaking teaching programs in mindful practice, communication skills, the patient-physician relationship, physician self-awareness, and the evaluation of professional competence.

V

Impact of Rochester's Biopsychosocial Education on Patient Care Skills

When medical school applicants arrive for interviews, they are immediately introduced to the BPS culture of the school. A large painting of George Engel hangs in the admissions area, and the associate dean for admissions emphasizes the curriculum's BPS underpinnings in his remarks at the beginning of applicants' interview days. In addition, the medical school's website mentions the BPS model prominently. Rochester graduates consistently rank the BPS orientation of their education highly on the Association of American Medical Colleges graduation questionnaire. Residency program directors give the patient communication skills of Rochester graduates high marks.[1] Over the last thirty years, a number of faculty members and associate deans at other medical schools have asked David Lambert and Jules Cohen, when they served as senior associate dean for medical education, "What do you *do* there? Your graduates who are here for residency training are *so* good at interacting with patients."[2] In clinical settings, former students have been praised with comments such as, "You must be a Rochester graduate."

Such feedback has led investigators to pose the following question: Do Rochester medical school graduates have patient care skills that flow from their BPS training? In 2000 Epstein and his colleagues conducted a large, year-long study of community-based physicians recruited from lists of all practicing physicians in Rochester. The researchers examined physician-patient communication by analyzing 197 audiotaped physician-patient encounters. Using a standardized communication analysis tool, the Rotor Interaction

Analysis System, they assessed the association between physician communication skills and patient trust, patient satisfaction, physician satisfaction, health outcomes, and health care costs. When the data were analyzed (without prior knowledge of the physicians' medical schools of origin), the subset of physicians who reported being Rochester medical school graduates was found to have more highly developed patient-centered communication skills than others, on average.[3]

In a separate study, Elaine Dannefer, a Rochester-trained education researcher based in the medical school, collaborated with Jules Cohen to study whether Rochester medical school graduates had greater patient-centered and patient sensitivity skills.[4] Working with two anthropology graduate student observers serving as research assistants over two summers, Dannefer and Cohen conducted an observational study of twenty pediatric residents one summer and twenty internal medicine residents the next summer. In each case, half of the residents were Rochester graduates who would have had exposure to biopsychosocially oriented faculty in pediatrics and medicine—as well as to the overall BPS culture of the school.[5] The anthropologists worked from a standardized protocol for assessing residents' skills in the areas of interviewing, physical examination of patients, and patient and family communication and support skills. Each resident was observed multiple times in both outpatient and inpatient settings and was also interviewed personally. The investigators were blinded to the residents' medical schools of origin until the research observations had been completed and the data analyzed. The results showed that the residents who had attended medical school at Rochester were better at listening to patients and families, obtaining social and psychological information, providing empathic responses, and using nonverbal comforting behaviors.[6] Further, even before the schools of origin were revealed, the anthropologist researchers had been able to identify *without error* which residents were Rochester graduates.

Both the Epstein and Dannefer data sets are relatively small and could be skewed if students who are themselves more biopsychosocially oriented choose to enroll at Rochester for their medical school training. Indeed, many applicants indicate that Rochester's BPS orientation is one of the bases for their interest in the school, as are its programs in student community service, international medicine, and medical humanities—which are rooted, at least in part, in the BPS philosophy. While the more biopsychosocially aware might choose Rochester initially, it can be argued that the Rochester environment fosters the more highly developed patient-centered skills they seek and exposes them to biopsychosocially oriented faculty who demonstrate and encourage the development of those skills. Further, the observational data overwhelmingly support the medical school's BPS impact on physician and resident behavior; self-selection bias is an unlikely explanation for these results. At the least, attending Rochester's medical school doesn't diminish the humanistic sensitivities many matriculants bring to their studies, as has been suggested in relation to some other medical schools.[7] In data collected on students at over seventy institutions, the Arnold P. Gold Foundation found that Rochester students are "off the page" relative to those at other schools, according to Sandra Gold, president and CEO of the foundation. According to the foundation's data, many more of Rochester's graduates come to medical school and leave it with a humanistic orientation. Gold commented to Jules Cohen, "At least you don't erode it the way they do at many other places."[8]

VI

Evolution of Research in Biopsychosocial Medicine at Rochester

When the Medical-Psychiatric Liaison Unit and Fellowship and the later Division of Behavioral and Psychosocial Medicine were operating and vital, individual faculty—following in Engel's footsteps—continued the tradition of pursuing observational studies of the role of psychological factors in various clinical diseases. In addition, interdepartmental collaborations, including those between medical school faculty and faculty in the liberal arts college, expanded the range of studies by rigorously applying the disciplines of philosophy, history, sociology, and psychology as well.

After Robert Ader was appointed director in 1982, the focus of the division's research moved in new directions.[1] Ader, who trained in experimental psychology, was a very highly regarded and productive researcher and a pioneer in studies of the effects of psychological stress on immune function.[2] He coined the term *psychoneuroimmunology* to identify this field of study and became a leader in the field. He was the founder and past president of the Psychoneuroimmunology Research Society, past president of the Academy of Behavioral Medicine Research and the American Psychosomatic Society, and he launched the journal *Brain, Behavior and Immunity*, which attracted many related papers. In a seminal study in the 1970s he and Nicholas Cohen, in the Department of Microbiology and Immunology, observed a kind of reverse placebo effect that showed a link between the brain and the immune system.[3] Rats had been given sweetened water along with an injection of Cytoxan, an immunosuppressive drug that causes stomach distress. After the Cytoxan injections were discontinued, the rats that had experienced stomach distress refused to drink the sweetened water. Ader and Cohen force-fed them the water, and some of the rats died. The taste of the sweetened water had stimulated neurological activity that suppressed their immune systems, just as if they had been overexposed to the Cytoxan, and the rats died of infections their immune systems couldn't handle. Ader and Cohen collaborated for many years and extended this work to include studies of the placebo effect in treatment of patients with psoriasis. Ader's highly respected work in Rochester and his influence there and elsewhere led to his designation as Distinguished University Professor and to other national and international honors, including an honorary medical degree from the University of Trondheim, an honorary Doctor of Science degree from Tulane University, and the Psychoneuroimmunology Research Society's creation of the Robert Ader New Investigator Award.

In 1981 Ader's *Psychoneuroimmunology* was first published, a classic text of writings in the field, which he compiled and edited.[4] Later editions were expanded by Ader and coeditors Nicholas Cohen and David Felten.[5] Felten, in the Department of Neurobiology and Anatomy, was also central to research in psychoneuroimmunology at Rochester.[6] Reinforcing the concept of a link between the immune and nervous systems, he demonstrated *anatomical* connections between the nervous system and immune cells. Felten was also able to show morphologic evidence of the autonomic innervations of spleen and lymph nodes with connections to T-cell receptors, affecting release of catecholamines, with effects on immune function. When Felten presented this work at a URMC conference in the late 1980s, Engel rose to say that he felt highly encouraged and that this was the direction research should be taking to illuminate basic mechanisms of mind-body processes.

The work of Ader, Cohen, and Felten thus documented the impact of psychological influences on the immune response, the behavioral conditioning of immune responses, and links between mental health (e.g., depression), levels of endogenous immune modulators, and subsequent illness.

A rich and diverse program of biopsychosocially related research, both clinical and basic, is still being pursued at the URMC. This research is based largely in the Departments of Psychiatry and

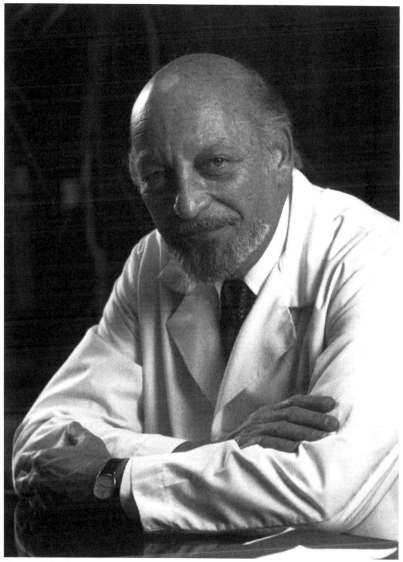

Figure 8. Robert Ader, 1989

Family Medicine and in the General Medicine Unit of the Department of Medicine. A leading BPS researcher in the General Medicine Unit is Geoffrey Williams, who has collaborated with Rochester psychologists Edward Deci and Richard Ryan on pioneering research applying self-determination theory and practice to motivation for smoking cessation, dietary modification, and diabetic management.[7] Their work incorporates biopsychosocially oriented interviewing, counseling, and patient care and requires excellent physician-patient communication skills. Collaborative research coming out of the General Medicine Unit and the Department of Family Medicine by Epstein, Krasner, Quill, Suchman, and others measures beneficial effects of mind-body stress reduction (MBSR).[8] A separate but related study by Jan Moynihan and Paul Duberstein has examined the effects of MBSR on immune responses, psychological well-being, and physical health in older adults.[9] In other collaborative work, Diane Morse—working with McDaniel, Epstein, and Elizabeth Edwardsen—has studied patient-physician communication in general practice, domestic violence, and cancer settings and is now studying self-determination theory as applied to medical problems of women with comorbid substance abuse, trauma, and criminal justice involvement.[10] Gary Morrow leads a team concerned with psychological issues in patients with cancer, not unrelated to Arthur Schmale's earlier work on factors important in the precipitation and course of malignancy.[11]

The Department of Psychiatry has continued Romano's pioneering advocacy for biopsychosocially oriented research through the ongoing strong support of department chair Eric Caine;[12] the leadership of Jan Moynihan, who directs the NIH-supported Rochester Center for Mind-Body Research; and the work of others.[13] Other biopsychosocially oriented research in the Department of Psychiatry includes studies of the impact of personality and stress on various disease states, including physiological and cognitive disease activity in multiple sclerosis;[14] the role of psychological factors in disease manifestation in psoriasis, eczema, and atopic dermatitis;[15] the medical and psychological needs and outcomes in patients undergoing dialysis;[16] and the effects of mindfulness treatment on clinical outcomes of psoriasis.[17] In addition, Catherine Cerulli is leading scholarly work in the Laboratory for Interpersonal Violence and Victimization,[18] and a bourgeoning group of researcher-clinicians is conducting health services and interventional research in court settings (such as mental health and drug treatment courts), addressing issues including motivation for treatment, substance abuse, and health services utilization.[19]

VII

National and International Scene

Although Rochester remains a focus of the BPS tradition, the approach has expanded across the United States and internationally to, for example, Australia, Canada, China, England, Finland, France, Israel, the Netherlands, Norway, and Switzerland. In large part, these developments have evolved from the dissemination of BPS principles by individuals who have had direct connections with Rochester, Engel, or Romano. Their research and teaching interests include the centrally important area of patient-physician communication, as well as motivation, somatization or medically unexplained symptoms, domestic violence, HIV communication issues, patient and physician satisfaction, trust, cost of care, ethnicity, economic and racial disparities in care, end-of-life care, physician self-disclosure, cancer communication strategies, and psychoneuroimmunology. Although Engel may not have enumerated each of these areas of interest when he originally described the BPS model, many who care for patients have come to understand the central role such psychosocial factors play in patient care.

The work of four former Rochester liaison fellows provides examples. At the University of North Carolina, Douglas Drossman established a highly regarded consultation liaison program in the Gastroenterology Clinic. Drossman found substantial evidence that patients with psychosomatic symptoms benefit from a broad, patient-centered BPS approach to their diagnosis and treatment.[1] He is now president of the Rome Foundation, playing important national and international roles in BPS medicine.

Mack Lipkin, the director of primary care internal medicine at New York University School of Medicine, is a leading researcher in the field of physician-patient communication and the founding president of what is now the American Academy on Communication in Healthcare (AACH). He developed the Lipkin Model, which teaches biopsychosocially related knowledge, skills, and attitudes in intensive workshops that influence the behavior of students, residents, and practitioners.[2]

Dennis Novack has become recognized for a career of teaching and research in physician-patient communication and psychosocial aspects of care. He has directed psychosocially oriented programs for residents and medical students at the University of Virginia, Brown University, and now Drexel University, where he directs clinical skills teaching and assessment, as well as the first-year course on physician-patient communication, psychosocial aspects of care, and physician personal awareness and well-being. Novack has been very active for many years in the AACH (discussed later) and the American Psychosomatic Society, serving as its president in 2002–3. In 2012 the Society of General Internal Medicine presented him with the National Award for Career Achievements in Medical Education for a lifetime of contributions to medical education.

At the University of Bern in Switzerland, former Engel fellow Rolf Adler has been teaching a clinical seminar for medical students based on the Morgan and Engel book *The Clinical Approach to the Patient*, as well as training residents in programs based on the BPS approach. The semistructured patient interview Engel advocated has been central to this effort, and the University of Bern awarded Engel an honorary MD in 1980. Adler and his colleagues have also been active in the American Psychosomatic Society and have written extensively about the BPS approach.[3] His successor at Bern, Roland von Kaenel, continues the work and also serves on the editorial board of *Psychosomatic Medicine*. Elsewhere around the world, other former Rochester liaison fellows, medical student fellows, and their associates have been involved in education and research projects in many areas of BPS interest.[4]

The AACH is another expression of the Engel-Romano legacy.[5] Composed almost entirely of primary care physicians who support biopsychosocially oriented teaching and research, this organization was cofounded by Mack Lipkin and Sam Putnam, another former Engel fellow.[6] At the first meeting of the Society for Research and Education in Primary Care Internal Medicine (SREPCIM) in 1978, they announced their intentions to start a task force focused on physician-patient communication. Among those interested was Dennis Novack, who became deeply involved in the organization. So did a number of other internists, many of whom were also graduates of Rochester's liaison fellowship—including Drossman, Suchman, and Quill.

The AACH sponsors six-day courses, both nationally and internationally, which include large-group demonstration interviews, observed medical interviews with detailed feedback, and personal awareness and family-of-origin small groups.[7] Putnam and Lipkin developed a style of active self-learning experiences for the small groups. These small-group experiences further the BPS principles of patient-physician communication and are applicable to clinical teaching rounds and other active learning formats, such as problem-based learning in the basic sciences. Novack codirected some of the early AACH faculty development programs and has taught in many of the organization's annual courses for more than twenty years. The influence of Romano and Engel is felt in the following approach of their former trainees: "Let the patient talk; listen, hear, and understand."[8]

The AACH research conferences have featured topics including Health Literacy, Innovative Strategies for Patient Education and Counseling, and a variety of other issues in physician-patient communication. Every year the group presents the Engel Research Award for Outstanding Research Contributing to the Theory, Practice, and Teaching of Effective Health Care Communication and Related Skills. Award recipients have included Engel, Epstein, Frankel, Wendy Levinson, Lipkin, Putnam, and Williams.

In many cases, the Romano-Engel influence has extended to individuals who were not trained at Rochester but who have become leaders in the expanding field of BPS medicine and developed their work more independently. One notable example is Shimon Glick, an internist at Ben Gurion University, who is professor emeritus, former chair of medicine, founder of the Israeli Society of Medical Ethics, and a pioneering researcher and teacher in BPS medicine.[9] Although he did not train at Rochester, Glick emulated Engel after meeting him and reading his writings many years ago. Glick has been instrumental in a biopsychosocially oriented medical education program at Ben Gurion, where he has also been involved in several studies documenting medical student skills in patient care.[10] The program at Ben Gurion teaches students to be aware of the psychological and social components, as well as the medical aspects, of their patients' problems—and to acknowledge that these family, community, and cultural factors are important in health and illness. This Engel-inspired program produces physicians seen as among the most sensitive and sophisticated communicators and medical communication educators throughout Israel.[11] Also in Israel, family physician Shmuel Reis, based in Bar-Ilan University's Faculty of Medicine in Galilee, is an internationally known researcher and educator in BPS medicine who has collaborated with Morse, McDaniel, and Epstein at the URMC.

At McMaster University in Canada, the BPS aspects of medical education are evident in several of the school's stated objectives: "The competent graduate recognizes the diverse factors that influence the health of the individual and the community; identifies the sociocultural, familial, psychological, economic, environmental, legal, political and spiritual factors impacting health care and health care delivery; and responds to these factors by planning and advocating the appropriate course of action at both the individual and the community level."[12]

In the United States, the influence of Romano and Engel can also be found in curricular mandates from the Institute of Medicine (IOM). Nine US medical schools were awarded behavioral and social sciences demonstration projects centered in primary care programs (general medicine units and family medicine) and received NIH funding for measuring outcomes of integrated four-year curricula they developed as a result of these mandates, which include

1. integrated curricula, across both preclinical and clinical years;
2. comprehensive assessment of behavioral and social science competencies;
3. clearly defined faculty development in IOM-required content domains; and
4. definition of the learning environment, with attention to the "hidden curriculum" with regard to the behavioral and social sciences.[13]

Although the BPS model has spread to many institutions, there is a risk of complacency about its place in medical education. Because so many US medical students and residents are taught about physician-patient communication, there is an assumption that these BPS strategies will later be incorporated into patient care. However, multiple recent analyses of audiotaped clinical interactions reveal that this is not consistently the case.[14]

Even at Rochester, with the glut of information students and residents encounter, as well as faculty assumptions that the BPS model is "probably being taught elsewhere" in the curriculum, less time is allotted for BPS teaching than was the case in Engel and Romano's era. This situation risks making students and residents sort out the application of these principles for themselves as they see them practiced instead of systematically learning BPS strategies.

Still, Rochester remains a place unlike any other. BPS medicine is said to be "in the air we breathe."[15] Interested faculty and students are drawn here as a result, further reinforcing Rochester's BPS culture. Moynihan notes, "Everywhere you go, Rochester is associated with Romano and Engel."[16] Epstein notes that the legacy of BPS medicine *has to be* in Rochester because, although Rochester may not lead in all aspects of biopsychosocially related research, there is a "special, nonspecific way" Rochester is different in research, education, and clinical care.[17] When Morse was choosing among three US BPS fellowships in 1990, her mentor Wendy Levinson advised her that Rochester was the best choice because it was "the Mecca of biopsychosocial medicine."[18] The BPS model and the ongoing tension between it and the biomedical model are even felt in student humor. A Rochester medical school T-shirt proclaimed, "I am a Biopsychosocialist," and a comic skit in a school play portrayed a critically ill patient being sensitively interviewed instead of being moved expeditiously to the operating room.

If Engel and Romano were at the University of Rochester School of Medicine today, they would certainly see that much has changed and would have much to suggest. Yet they would also find much to admire and would be proud of how much their strong influence remains in medicine today, both at Rochester and elsewhere—especially considering the pressures of the current practice environment that make the BPS approach to the patient more difficult.

VIII

Current Views of the Biopsychosocial Model

Since Engel's landmark article in 1977 and subsequent expansions, the BPS model has become widely accepted as a useful contribution to medicine and medical education worldwide.[1] For over thirty years, scholars have written widely about the model, both praising and criticizing it. They have endeavored to clarify its meaning and role in clinical practice, defined its content for medical curricula, viewed it in the context of their experiences with Engel the man, tried to place it in the context of systems thinking, questioned Engel's claim of original thinking in authorship, and attempted to empirically prove or disprove its validity as a way of explaining disease processes. Many graduates of Rochester's medical school, residencies, or liaison fellowship, as well as faculty, have coauthored such writings.

In support of the impact of the BPS model in practice, primary care physicians Francesc Borrell-Carrio, Anthony Suchman, and Ronald Epstein noted in 2004 that it is a "philosophy of clinical care and a practical clinical guide."[2] They defended the model's scientific foundation and the framework of complexity theory Engel used to view disease causes as multifactorial and reciprocal rather than linear. They also suggested clarifications to the model and strategies for operationalizing it in clinical practice, including physician self-awareness, establishment of a calibrated clinician-patient partnership, and application of medical knowledge in a patient-centered fashion.

In contrast, psychiatrist Herbert Weiner wrote in 1994 that Engel's systems-theory-based model, developed to "order the world from the most elementary particles to social phenomena and the cosmos," is obsolete because of feedback between the different levels and because it is a reductionist explanation of complexity, order, and change.[3] While it is true that systems and complexity theories are core principles of the BPS model, a claim that the model is no longer useful seems somewhat reductionist itself, since Weiner does not address the patient-physician communication that is so fundamental to the model or acknowledge Engel's key role in synthesizing and disseminating it. Engel's writings on the systems approach acknowledge the importance of interactions between different rungs of the BPS ladder, also noted by Borrell-Carrio and colleagues.[4]

In another paper that addresses dualistic debates over pharmacologic versus psychotherapeutic psychiatric approaches using the BPS model as a rationale to reject medication, psychiatrist Edward Shorter noted in 2005 that the "therapeutic use of the doctor-patient relationship . . . is precisely the message that the biopsychosocial model has for us today." He opined that the "biopsychosocial model failed to catch on" because of the coincident "stunning success of pharmacotherapy" in the late twentieth century. He countered, however, that "post-modern medicine" has revealed "the weaknesses of the pharmacological approach" and that current medicine has a "much greater receptiveness to non-pharmacological approaches, . . . especially to functional" problems. Interestingly, Shorter specifically mentions others, such as Adolph Meyer, who influenced Engel's views. But he maintains that Engel should be credited as the one who brought the concepts together and "placed the biopsychosocial model firmly on the undergraduate teaching agenda of the world's medical schools and on the educational programme of residency training in psychiatry in many places." Further, Shorter dismisses Meyer's views as "nothing more than an accumulation of the platitudes of the day," implying that Engel's contribution took Meyer's views to a unique and new level.[5]

As part of a 2002 Australian symposium on Engel's contribution to psychiatry, psychiatrist Graeme Taylor critically reviewed the body of Engel's work. He concluded that Engel had "successfully bridged the disciplines of medicine, psychiatry, and psychoanalysis and broadened the scope of psychosomatic research and clinical practice by identifying the role of interpersonal relationships . . . in regulating mental and bodily processes."[6]

A uniquely mixed opinion came in 2002 from Bruce Singh, a psychiatrist who also participated in the Australian psychiatric symposium and who wrote a "personal reminiscence" in response to an editor's request after Engel's death in 1999. In it he described a number of negative impressions of Engel's research and teaching methods from his time as a liaison fellow with Engel in 1975–77. A number of Singh's difficulties had to do with Engel insisting on his own identity and skills as an internist and declining what he saw as strictly psychiatric work. Mack Lipkin, whose time overlapped that of Singh, made similar comments about Engel's inability or unwillingness to supervise more specifically psychiatric cases.[7] Another possible reason Engel persistently avoided gaining expertise in psychiatry might have been to distinguish himself as an internist and thus advance his view that nonpsychiatrists should also have advanced communication skills. Despite his criticisms, Singh wrote that he incorporates the BPS approach in his own teaching and concluded that Engel will be remembered as a "medical Darwin."[8]

In addition to Singh, several other critics have raised issues about the BPS model. For example, Niall A. McLaren questions whether it is, in fact, a "model," as models are traditionally defined scientifically.[9] Further, in a 2009 article, Hamid Tavakoli suggests that the BPS model creates an artificial distinction between biology and psychology.[10] It is notable that several of the more negative perspectives on the BPS model come from the psychiatric literature. There is still, however, strong support from multiple disciplines for the model's relevance to clinical practice and its role as a foundation for the type of research done by Douglas Drossman, George Engel, William Greene, Mack Lipkin, Arthur Schmale, Bing-Jiun Shen, Andrew Steptoe, and others.[11]

The role of the BPS model in medical school teaching was discussed by Dennis Novack in an article based on his presidential address at the annual meeting of the American Psychosomatic Society in March 2003. Novack outlined a clinical and research-based rationale for integrating psychosomatic medicine into medical curricula, described current educational deficiencies in such curricula, and proposed a detailed core curriculum and strategies for its implementation. In support of the BPS model, he asserted, "The field of psychosomatic medicine is vibrant, exciting, and young" and described ongoing publication of "important new research that advances our understanding of how mind/brain/body and social context interact in health and in illness."[12] He concluded: "There has never been a more propitious time for influencing the next generation of physician scientists and practitioners than now. I believe that, with our collegial and determined efforts, we can all contribute to realizing Engel's vision. With the integration of psychosomatic medicine into medical curricula, medical schools will begin graduating physicians who can heal as well as they can cure, practicing their craft within a biopsychosocial model of care."[13]

This message of hope for the role of the BPS model and medical education is shared by many other leaders in the field. Since the groundbreaking work of Engel and Romano, the model has evolved and grown. The extraordinarily rich legacy of these two men will continue to illuminate our understanding of health, illness, and the practice of medicine, benefiting future generations of physicians and their patients.

Notes

Chapter One

1. Theodore M. Brown, "The Historical and Conceptual Foundations of the Rochester Biopsychosocial Model," *Human Nature Review*, accessed June 22, 2011, http://human-nature.com/free-associations/engel2.html; and Jules Cohen and Stephanie Brown Clark, *John Romano and George Engel: Their Lives and Work* (Rochester, NY: University of Rochester Press, 2010). Theodore Brown is professor of history, public health sciences, and medical humanities, and the Charles E. and Dale L. Phelps Professor of Public Health and Policy at Rochester.

2. John Romano to Eugene Ferris, February 18, 1942, box 8, folder 10, John Romano Papers, Edward G. Miner Library, University of Rochester Medical Center, Rochester, NY.

3. George L. Engel, "From Biomedical to Biopsychosocial II: A Personal Odyssey," *Families, Systems, & Health* 14, no. 4 (1996): 447–48.

Chapter Two

1. Jules Cohen, "George L. Engel, MD," *Journal of the American Medical Association* 283, no. 21 (2001): 2857. The course textbook was George L. Engel, *Psychological Development in Health and Disease* (Philadelphia: W. B. Saunders, 1962).

2. Brown, "Historical and Conceptual Foundations."

3. George L. Engel, "The Need for a New Medical Model: A Challenge for Biomedicine," *Science* 196 (1977): 129–36.

4. Arthur H. Schmale, William A. Greene, Franz Reichsman, M. Kehoe, and George L. Engel, "An Established Program of Graduate Education in Psychosomatic Medicine," *Advances in Psychosomatic Medicine* 4 (1964): 4–13.

5. William L. Morgan and George L. Engel, *The Clinical Approach to the Patient* (Philadelphia: W. B. Saunders, 1969).

6. Laurence Guttmacher, interview by Diane Morse and Jules Cohen, July 2, 2008. David H. Rosen was associate professor of psychiatry and medicine at Rochester 1982–86. He received his MD from the University of Missouri (Columbia) and did psychiatric training at the Langley Porter Institute (University of California Medical Center, San Francisco), where he served on the faculty until 1982. He is the McMillan Professor of Analytical Psychology and professor of humanities in medicine and of psychiatry and behavioral science at Texas A&M University.

7. Jules Cohen, Sharon K. Krackov, Edgar R. Black, and Mary-Margaret Holyst, "Introduction to Human Health and Illness: A Series of Patient-Centered Conferences Based on the Biopsychosocial Model," *Academic Medicine* 75, no. 4 (2000): 390–96.

8. Laurence Guttmacher received his MD from Case Western Reserve University. At Rochester, he is clinical professor of psychiatry and medical humanities, as well as associate dean, advising.

9. Laurence Guttmacher, informal conversation with Jules Cohen, July 2008.

10. Kathryn Markakis, interview by Morse, June 2007.

11. Ibid.

Chapter Three

1. Timothy Quill, interview by Cohen, August 2005. Nancy S. Clark received her MD from the University of Rochester. She completed a residency in internal medicine at the URMC's Strong Memorial Hospital and a fellowship in geriatric medicine at Monroe Community Hospital in Rochester. She is clinical assistant professor of medicine at Rochester. Eric Richard graduated from Yale School of Medicine, did his residency training in Rochester, and is assistant professor of medicine at Rochester. Timothy Quill is a University of Rochester medical school graduate who served as a resident in the institution's Primary Care Program in Internal Medicine and as a liaison fellow in 1979–81. He holds joint appointments as professor of medicine and psychiatry and directs the Palliative Care Program at Rochester.

2. Markakis and Eric Richard, e-mail messages to Morse, June 2007.

3. Kathryn Markakis, general internist, is a graduate of Wayne State Medical School. At Rochester, she did her residency in the Primary Care Program in Internal Medicine and the liaison fellowship in 1988. She is associate professor of clinical medicine at Rochester. Anthony Suchman received his MD from Cornell University. He was a resident in Roches-

ter's Primary Care Program in Internal Medicine and then one of Engel's liaison fellows. He went on to codirect and teach in the later version of the liaison fellowship in the late 1980s and early 1990s and is now actively involved in student and resident teaching. He is clinical professor of medicine at Rochester and administers Leading Organizations to Health, a program promoting relationship-centered health care through organizational change. Anne Nofziger is associate professor of family medicine at Rochester. She received her MD from Indiana University School of Medicine. She did a family medicine residency and two years as chief resident at Rochester, joined the faculty in 2000, and completed a Dean's Teaching Fellowship in 2007, with a project focusing on peer assessment.

4. Preclinical medical students at the URMC, personal conversation with Jules Cohen, October 2011.

5. Michael Krasner is a 1987 graduate of UC San Diego Medical School and the Rochester medicine-pediatrics residency program. He is associate professor of clinical medicine at Rochester, a practitioner of mindfulness-based stress reduction, and offers a related seminar to first- and second-year students as part of the medical humanities electives. This method is based on meditation and mindful Hatha Yoga and has applications to everyday life. It was initially developed by Jon Kabat-Zinn.

6. Dennis Novack, interview by Morse, June 2007; Douglas Drossman, interview by Morse and Cohen, June 2007.

7. David A. Davis, Mary Ann Thompson, Andrew D. Oxman, and R. Brian Hayes, "Changing Physician Performance: A Systematic Review of the Effect of Continuing Medical Education Strategies," *Journal of the American Medical Association* 274 (1995): 700–705.

8. Milatti Srinivasin, Peter Franks, Lisa S. Meredith, Kevin Fiscella, Ronald M. Epstein, and Richard L. Kravitz, "Connoisseurs of Care? Unannounced Standardized Patients' Ratings of Physicians," *Medical Care* 44 (2006): 1092–98; Kevin Fiscella, Peter Franks, Milatti Srinivasin, Richard L. Kravitz, and Ronald M. Epstein, "Ratings of Physician Communication by Real and Standardized Patients," *Annals of Family Medicine* 5, no. 2 (2007): 151–58.

9. Ralph F. Jozefowicz, professor of neurology and medicine, received his MD from Columbia University College of Physicians and Surgeons in 1979. He completed residencies in internal medicine and neurology, as well as a fellowship in neuromuscular diseases at Rochester. Jeffrey M. Lyness received his MD with honor and with distinction in research from the University of Rochester in 1986. He completed an internship in internal medicine there and a psychiatry residency at Yale, prior to returning to Rochester for clinical and research fellowships in geriatric psychiatry. He also did a fellowship with the National Cancer Institute on motivation and

4As counseling for tobacco dependence, 1992–94. He is senior associate dean for academic affairs and professor of psychiatry at Rochester.

10. Valerie Lang received her MD from SUNY Upstate Medical Center. She has been an internal medicine hospitalist at Rochester since 2000 and is associate professor of medicine. She directs the third-year Adult Inpatient Medicine Clerkship, the Medicine Sub-Internship, and the Hospital Medicine Faculty Development program.

11. The term *stress* as used in this context is totally distinct from its usage in Hans Selye, "Stress and Disease," *Science* 122 (1955): 625–31. In this present context, "stress reduction" applies to the relief of psychological processes such as anxiety, depression, and the like, which affect patients' health and illness, as understood by Engel, Romano, and their colleagues—as well as present-day biopsychosocially oriented physicians.

12. Markakis, interview; Ronald Epstein, interview by Morse, June 2007; Jan Moynihan, interview by Morse and Cohen, June 2007.

13. See Romano's CV in appendix to Cohen and Brown Clark, *John Romano and George Engel.*

14. Kathryn Montgomery received a PhD in literature from Emory University and was initially appointed to the Department of Preventive, Family, and Rehabilitation Medicine at Rochester. Her primary appointment changed to the Division of the Medical Humanities once the division was established. She is now professor of medical humanities and bioethics and of medicine at Northwestern School of Medicine in Chicago and director of the Master of Arts in Medical Humanities and Bioethics graduate program there.

15. Jane Greenlaw received her JD and MSN degrees from Boston College after obtaining her RN from New England Baptist Hospital. Before retiring in 2012, she was associate professor of the medical humanities, directed the Ethics Consultation Service at Strong Memorial Hospital, taught law and ethics to medical students and residents, and served on the New York State Task Force on Life and the Law.

16. Marjorie Hodges Shaw is assistant professor in the Division of Bioethics. She received an MA in philosophy from the University of Rochester, a JD from Cornell Law School, and a PhD from the University of Rochester's Warner School of Education in 2011.

17. Stephanie Brown Clark is associate professor of the medical humanities; a graduate of McMaster School of Medicine in Hamilton, Ontario, Canada; and holds doctorates in English literature and medical history from the University of Leiden in the Netherlands. For a number of years, she also chaired Rochester's George W. Corner Society for the History of Medicine, composed of faculty, practicing physicians, residents, students,

and others interested in the field who meet monthly during the academic year to hear presentations about topics related to the history of medicine.

18. For example, Mindy Shah, Timothy Quill, Sally Norton, Yvonne Sada, Marcia Buckley, and Charlotte Fridd, "What Bothers You the Most? Initial Responses from Patients Receiving Palliative Care Consultation," *American Journal of Hospice and Palliative Medicine* 25 (2008): 88–92; Timothy Quill, "Terri Schiavo: A Tragedy Compounded," *New England Journal of Medicine* 352 (2005): 16–21; Quill, interview.

19. Thomas Campbell, interview by Morse, June 2007. Interestingly, Romano served as a mentor for Campbell during his fellowship because Engel was recovering from bypass surgery. According to Campbell, Romano championed the importance of research into the central role of the family in health and illness and was instrumental in mentoring Campbell's later research. Epstein, interview; Susan McDaniel, interview by Morse, June 2007.

20. Engel, conversations with liaison fellow Morse and others, early 1990s. Over the years, Rochester medical students and fellows saw and learned from movies (converted to videotapes) made during the Monica studies. Significant understandings about basic psychobiological principles arose from this work on the concept of conservation withdrawal. These valuable tapes now reside at Harvard University.

21. McDaniel, interview.

22. For example, John Romano, Robert H. Geertsma, and S. S. Trieshmann, "Studies of Schizophrenic Parents and the Caretaking Process: Work in Progress," in *Georgian M. Asatiani Research Institute of Psychiatry, Fiftieth Anniversary Jubilee*, vols. 21–22 (Tbilisi, USSR: 1976): 208–13.

23. Diane Morse, "An Interview with George Engel, M.D.," *Families, Systems, & Health* 14, no. 4 (1996): 413–24.

24. George L. Engel, "From Biomedical to Biopsychosocial I: Being Scientific in the Human Domain," *Families, Systems, & Health* 14, no. 4 (1996): 425–33; Engel, "From Biomedical to Biopsychosocial II," 434–49.

Chapter Four

1. William A. Greene Jr., Lawrence E. Young, and Scott N. Swisher, "Psychological Factors and Reticuloendothelial Disease, Part I," *Psychosomatic Medicine* 16 (1954): 220–30; William A. Greene Jr., "Role of a Vicarious Object in the Adaptation to Object Loss, Part I," *Psychosomatic Medicine* 20 (1958): 344–50; William A. Greene Jr., "Role of a Vicarious Object in the Adaptation to Object Loss, Part II," *Psychosomatic Medicine* 21 (1959): 438–47.

2. William A. Greene Jr., Sidney Goldstein, and Arthur J. Moss, "Psychological Aspects of Sudden Death: A Preliminary Report," *Archives of Internal Medicine* 129, no. 5 (1972): 725–31.

3. Arthur H. Schmale Jr., "Relationship of Separation and Depression to Disease," *Psychosomatic Medicine* 20 (1958): 259–77.

4. George L. Engel and Arthur H. Schmale Jr., "The Psychoanalytic Theory of Somatic Disorder: Conversion, Specificity, and the Disease Onset Situation," *Journal of the American Psychoanalytic Association* 15 (1967): 344–65; Arthur H. Schmale Jr. and Howard P. Iker, "Hopelessness as a Predictor of Cervical Carcinoma," *Social Science and Medicine* 5 (1971): 95–100.

5. Sanford Meyerowitz, "The Continuing Investigation of Psychosocial Variables in Rheumatoid Arthritis," *Modern Trends in Rheumatology* 2 (1971): 92–105; Sanford Meyerowitz, "Psychological Factors in the Etiology of Somatic Disease," *Annals of Internal Medicine* 72, no. 5 (1970): 753–54; V. Mei-Tal, Sanford Meyerowitz, and George L. Engel, "The Role of Psychological Process in a Somatic Disorder: Multiple Sclerosis," *Psychosomatic Medicine* 32, no. 1 (1970): 67–86.

6. "The Rochester Plan," *Rochester Review* (Spring 1976): 26.

7. George L. Engel, Franz Reichsman, and Harry L. Segal, "A Study of an Infant with a Gastric Fistula: I. Behavior and the Rate of Total Hydrochloric Acid Secretion," *Psychosomatic Medicine* 18 (1956): 374–98; George L. Engel and Franz Reichsman, "Spontaneous and Experimentally Induced Depressions in an Infant with a Gastric Fistula: A Contribution to the Problem of Depression," *Journal of the American Psychoanalytic Association* 4 (1956): 428–52.

8. Drossman and Novack, interviews by Morse, June 2007; Mack Lipkin, interview by Morse and Cohen, June 2007.

9. Epstein, Novack, Drossman, and Lipkin, interviews.

10. Rolf Adler received his MD from the University of Bern, Switzerland. He was a liaison fellow at Rochester in 1967–69. He has retired from his position as professor of internal medicine and physician-in-chief in the Department of General Internal Medicine at Bern, but he is still involved in residency education and works part-time as an internist and a psychotherapist. Rolf Adler, personal letter to Jules Cohen, August 4, 2011. Douglas Drossman received his MD from Albert Einstein College of Medicine, completed his residency in medicine at the University of North Carolina at Chapel Hill (UNC), and did a tour of duty in Vietnam before coming to the liaison fellowship in 1975–76. He subsequently specialized in gastroenterology and has been an effective and productive investigator. His frequently cited, important work includes research into the association between somatization disorder and a history of childhood abuse; for example: Douglas A. Drossman, Jane

Lesserman, Ginette Nachman, Zhiming Li, Honi Gluck, Timothy Toomey, and Madeline Mitchell, "Sexual and Physical Abuse in Women with Functional or Organic Gastrointestinal Disorders," *Annals of Internal Medicine* 113, no. 11 (1990): 828–33. He served as professor of medicine and psychiatry and founder and codirector of the UNC Center for Functional GI and Motility Disorders. He is now an adjunct faculty member at UNC and president of the Rome Foundation. Ronald M. Epstein received his MD from Harvard Medical School and did his internship and residency in family medicine, as well as a 1984–85 fellowship in family medicine, psychiatry, and HIV, at Highland Hospital in Rochester. He is professor of family medicine, psychiatry, oncology, and nursing at the URMC. In addition to his clinical work, Epstein is director of the Center for Communication and Disparities Research, which focuses on how to improve communication among clinicians, patients, and their loved ones. He is also very active in medical education and educational research and is director of the Dean's Teaching Fellowship Program. Epstein has received the Lynn Payer Award from the American Academy on Communication in Healthcare for lifetime achievement in communication research. His various studies, funded by the NIH, the Agency for Healthcare Research and Quality, and various foundations, have focused on the effects patient-physician communications can have on patients' health, the process of care, and health care costs. Mack Lipkin received his MD from Harvard Medical School, went to UNC for his first two years of internal medicine residency, completed a third year at Rochester, and then entered the liaison fellowship in 1973. He is professor of medicine at New York University School of Medicine. Examples of publications are Mack Lipkin and Joshua Lee, *Clinical Addiction Psychiatry* (New York: Cambridge University Press, 2010); Sondra R. Zabar, Mack Lipkin, Kathleen Hanley, Angela Burgess, Julia Hyland Bruno, Jennifer G. Adams, Adina Kalet, and Colleen C. Gillespie, "Assessing Residents' Competence in Two Contexts: Standardized Patient Exams and Unannounced Standardized Patient Visits," *Journal of General Internal Medicine* 25, no. 9 (2010): 227. Dennis Novack graduated from Hahneman Medical College, completed an internal medicine residency at Bryn Mawr Hospital, and spent a year traveling before entering Rochester's liaison fellowship in 1976. He has been a leader in the AACH and played an important role in its founding. He is professor of medicine, associate dean of medical education, and director of clinical skills teaching and assessment at Drexel University College of Medicine.

11. Epstein, Lipkin, Novack, and Drossman, interviews.
12. Novack, interview.
13. Drossman, interview.
14. Novack, interview.
15. Lipkin and Novack, interviews.

16. Novack, Drossman, and Lipkin, interviews.

17. Lipkin and Novack, interviews.

18. Campbell, interview.

19. Thomas Campbell received his MD from Harvard. He completed residency training in family medicine at Rochester, as well as a liaison fellowship in behavioral and psychosocial medicine (1982–83). He is the William Rocktaschel Chair in Family Medicine and professor of family medicine and psychiatry at Rochester. He has written extensively on the relationship between families and health and has been coeditor of the journal *Families, Systems, & Health.*

20. At the time of his 2011 retirement until his death shortly thereafter, Robert Ader was Distinguished University Professor, Emeritus, at Rochester. His BS was from Tulane University, and he received a PhD in experimental psychology from Cornell University in 1957.

21. Theodore Brown, "George Engel and Rochester's Biopsychosocial Tradition: Historical and Developmental Perspectives," in *The Biopsychosocial Approach: Past, Present, Future,* ed. Richard Frankel, Timothy Quill, and Susan McDaniel (Rochester, NY: University of Rochester Press, 2003), 199–219; and telephone conversations between Cohen and Alvin L. Ureles, Rudolph J. Napodano, and Quill, August 2008. Cecile Carson is an MD graduate of the University of Texas Southwestern Medical School and the internal medicine residency program at Temple University. At Rochester, she was a liaison fellow in 1977–79 and a faculty member until 2006, most recently as clinical associate professor of medicine and psychiatry. For over twenty-five years she has focused much of her work on helping people deal with life-threatening illness, such as HIV and cancer. Currently a shamanic health practitioner, she works in counseling and teaching rather than primary care internal medicine. Geoffrey Williams received his MD from Wayne State University School of Medicine and was attracted to Rochester's residency program because of its BPS orientation. At Rochester, he completed a residency in internal medicine and a PhD in psychology in the area of motivation and self-determination. He was in Rochester's liaison fellowship in 1986–88. Engel carefully read and discussed his thesis with him and recognized that it was closely related to biopsychosocially oriented patient care. Williams is now professor of medicine, psychiatry, and psychology at Rochester and directs the university's Healthy Living Center in the community. He is an internationally recognized investigator in self-determination theory, important in behavioral change. Geoffrey Williams, interview by Morse and Cohen, June 2007.

22. Howard Beckman, former chief of medicine at Highland Hospital, an affiliate operated by the University of Rochester, is now medical director of the Rochester Independent Practice Association and clinical professor

of medicine at the university. Richard Frankel has left Rochester and is at Indiana University, where he is professor of medicine and geriatrics, senior research scientist at the Regenstrief Institute, and senior scientist at the Center for Implementing Evidence-Based Practice Health at the Richard L. Roudebush VA Medical Center. Beckman and Frankel's work involved teaching and research on the medical interview. In an often-cited paper, they reported studies of physicians frequently interrupting interviews, with the remarkable finding of an interval of only eighteen seconds before a patient was interrupted by his or her primary care physician. Howard Beckman and Richard M. Frankel, "The Effect of Physician Behavior on the Collection of Data," *Annals of Internal Medicine* 101 (1984): 692–96. Susan McDaniel is the Dr. Laurie Sands Distinguished Professor of Families and Health in the Departments of Psychiatry and Family Medicine and is associate chair of family medicine at Rochester. She has also been coeditor of the journal *Families, Systems, & Health.* She received a PhD from UNC in clinical psychology, did her internship at the University of Texas Medical Branch in Galveston, and was a fellow in family therapy at the Texas Research Institute for Mental Services in Houston. Before leaving the URMC in 2009, Richard Botelho was professor of family medicine at Rochester. He received his BMedSci from Nottingham Medical School and did a residency in family practice at Birmingham Heartlands Hospital, both in England.

23. Rudolph Napodano, personal conversation with Cohen, August 2008.

24. Betty Rabinowitz is a primary care physician who graduated from Ben Gurion University Medical School, where she also completed a residency in internal medicine. She completed Rochester's liaison fellowship in 1993 and is associate professor of clinical medicine and medical director of the URMC Center for Primary Care. Steven Novak received his MD from the University of Pittsburgh School of Medicine and is a graduate of Rochester's Family Medicine Residency Program. He is assistant professor of clinical psychiatry and of family medicine at the URMC and a lead investigator in substance abuse treatment. David N. Smith is a physician in private practice in Rochester. He completed medical school and a PhD in neuroanatomy at the URMC and holds a postdoctoral fellowship in neuro-ophthalmology from Harvard.

Chapter Five

1. David Lambert, interview by Morse and Cohen, May 2007.

2. Ibid. David Lambert received his MD from Dartmouth Medical School and completed residency training at Deaconess Hospital. At Roch-

ester, he is professor of medicine and senior associate dean for medical student education.

3. Epstein, e-mails to Morse regarding unpublished research, June 2007.

4. Elaine Dannefer received her PhD in sociology from the University of Rochester. She served for five years as associate dean for curricular affairs at the URMC and is now director of medical education research and assessment at the Cleveland Clinic Lerner College of Medicine, Case Western Reserve University.

5. For example, pediatrics faculty Elizabeth McAnarney, O. J. Sahler, and Richard Kreipe. McAnarney completed her MD and residency training at SUNY at Upstate Medical University, as well as a fellowship in adolescent medicine at URMC. She is professor and chair emerita of pediatrics. Sahler received her MD from Rochester and completed residency training at Duke and Rochester. She is professor of pediatrics, hematology, and oncology and of psychiatry and medical humanities. Kreipe received his MD from Tempie University, did residency training at St. Christopher's Hospital for Children, and completed a fellowship in adolescent medicine at Rochester. He is the Dr. Elizabeth R. McAnarney Professor in Pediatrics at URMC.

6. Elaine Dannefer and Jules Cohen, unpublished data, 1994.

7. A. Mohammadreca Hojat, Salvatore Mangione, Thomas J. Nasca, Susan Rattner, James B. Erdmann, Joseph S. Gonnella, and Mike Magee, "An Empirical Study of Decline in Empathy in Medical School," *Medical Education* 38 (2004): 934–41; Bruce W. Newton, Laurie Barber, James Clardy, Elton Cleveland, and Patricia O'Sullivan, "Is There a Hardening of the Heart During Medical School?" *Academic Medicine* 83 (2008): 244–49.

8. Sandra Gold, telephone conversation with Cohen, early 1990s.

Chapter Six

1. Lipkin and Campbell, interviews.

2. When Romano originally hired Ader in 1957, he had strong support from Engel, but some of the other clinically oriented faculty in psychiatry questioned the wisdom of appointing an experimental psychologist to the department. According to Ader, Romano responded, "Wait twenty years." Robert Ader, personal communication with Jules Cohen, April 11, 2005.

3. Robert Ader and Nicholas Cohen, "Behaviorally Conditioned Immunosuppression," *Psychosomatic Medicine* 37 (1975): 333–40. Before retiring, Nicholas Cohen was professor of microbiology and immunology and of

psychiatry at Rochester. He received his PhD from the University of Rochester in 1966.

4. Robert Ader, ed., *Psychoneuroimmunology* (New York: Academic Press, 1981).

5. Robert Ader, David L. Felten, and Nicholas Cohen, eds., *Psychoneuroimmunology*, 3rd ed. (San Diego: Academic Press, 2001).

6. David L. Felten received his MD and PhD from the University of Pennsylvania. He is vice president for research and medical director of the Beaumont Research Institute at the William Beaumont Hospitals in Royal Oak, MI.

7. Edward Deci is professor of psychology and Gowen Professor in the Social Sciences at the University of Rochester. After receiving his PhD from Carnegie Mellon University, he came to Rochester's Department of Psychology and developed the self-determination theory currently used and studied internationally in areas including business and medicine. He was joined by his former graduate student Richard Ryan, who received his PhD from the University of Rochester; together, they have continued to develop and study this model of behavioral change. Ryan is professor of psychology, psychiatry, and education at Rochester. Williams, interview.

8. These studies have been funded by the Arthur Vining Davis Foundation, the Physicians' Foundation for Health Systems Excellence, and Mannix, to assess the impact of MBSR training on the attitudes and behavior of medical students and primary care residents at Rochester.

9. Jan Moynihan received her PhD in microbiology from the University of Rochester School of Medicine and Dentistry. She is the Engel Professor in Psychosocial Medicine in the Department of Psychiatry and professor of microbiology and immunology at Rochester. She worked with Robert Ader and Nicholas Cohen in her graduate research on behavioral conditioning of immune responses, which Engel believed was a key offshoot of his work; Eric Caine (chair of psychiatry), personal communication with Cohen, January 19, 2005; Moynihan, interview. Paul Duberstein is professor of psychiatry and psychology at Rochester. He received his PhD in clinical psychology from SUNY Buffalo.

10. Elizabeth Edwardsen received her MD and completed a residency in internal medicine at Rochester. She is associate professor in emergency medicine at URMC.

11. Gary Morrow received his PhD from the University of Rhode Island in 1975. At Rochester, he is professor in the Departments of Radiation Oncology and Psychiatry and at the Wilmot Cancer Center.

12. Eric Caine is professor of psychiatry and neurology, chair of psychiatry, and the John Romano Professor of Psychiatry at Rochester. He

received his MD from Harvard Medical School and did residency training in psychiatry at Massachusetts Mental Health Center and the National Institute of Mental Health.

13. Moynihan, interview. Moynihan has researched stress-induced modulation of immune function, which Engel saw as a cutting-edge issue in BPS medicine.

14. Paul Duberstein, Andrew Goodman, and Raluca Topciu, co-PIs.

15. Duberstein and Francisco Tausk, co-PIs.

16. Moynihan, Quill, Duberstein, Williams, and Melissa Schiff, investigators.

17. Moynihan, McDonald, Tausk, and Ritchlin, co-PIs.

18. Catherine Cerulli received both her JD and PhD from the State University of New York at Albany. She is associate professor of psychiatry at Rochester.

19. Diane Morse, Marc Swogger, Catherine Cerulli, Steven Lamberti, and Geoffrey Williams.

Chapter Seven

1. Ingrid Pesetsky, Emily Keram, and Douglas A. Drossman, "Building a Psychiatric-Medical Liaison: Observations of the Process," *Psychiatric Medicine* 10, no. 2 (1992): 149–63.

2. Lipkin, interview; New York University Faculty Scholars Program; William Clark, Mack Lipkin, Howard Graman, and Jeannette Shorey, "Improving Physicians' Relationships with Patients," *Journal of General Internal Medicine* 14(S1) (1999): S45–S50.

3. Stefan M. Goetz, Marion Hahr, Thomas Koch, Christine Beer, Christof E. Minder, and Rolf H. Adler, "Characteristics of Fatigue of Psychogenic and Somatic Origin: Toward an Understanding of Different Manifestations of Fatigue," *Journal of Psychosomatic Research* 58 (2005): 179–82.

4. Diane S. Morse, Ross Lafleur, Colleen T. Fogarty, Mona Mittal, and Catherine Cerulli, "'They Told Me to Leave': How Health Care Providers Address Intimate Partner Violence," *Journal of the American Board of Family Medicine* 25, no. 3 (2012): 333–42; Diane S. Morse and Susan H. McDaniel, "Physicians, Relationships With," in *Encyclopedia of Human Relationships*, eds. Harry T. Reis and Susan K. Sprecher (Thousand Oaks, CA: Sage, 2009), 1252–55; Francesc Borrell-Carrio, Anthony L. Suchman, and Ronald M. Epstein, "The Biopsychosocial Model 25 Years Later: Principles, Practice, and Scientific Inquiry," *Annals of Family Medicine* 2 (2004): 576–82; Christine B. Dalton, Douglas A. Drossman, Joseph M. Hathaway, and Shrikant I. Bangdiwala, "Perceptions of Physicians and Patients with Organic and

Functional Gastrointestinal Diagnoses," *Clinical Gastroenterology and Hepatology* 2 (2004): 121–26; Ronald M. Epstein, Taj Hadee, Jennifer Carroll, Sean C. Meldrum, Judi Lardner, and Cleveland G. Shields, "Could This Be Something Serious? Reassurance, Uncertainty, and Empathy in Response to Patients' Expressions of Worry," *Journal of General Internal Medicine* 22, no. 12 (2007): 1731–39; Mitchell D. Feldman and John F. Christensen, eds., *Behavioral Medicine: A Guide for Clinical Practice*, 3rd ed. (New York: McGraw Hill, 2008); Stanford B. Friedman, Jules Cohen, and Howard Iker, "Antibody Response to Cholera Vaccine: Differences Between Depressed, Schizophrenic and Normal Subjects," *Archives of General Psychiatry* 16 (March 1967): 312–15; Mack Lipkin, Samuel M. Putnam, and Aaron Lazare, *The Medical Interview: Clinical Care, Education, and Research (New York: Springer-Verlag, 1995);* Diane S. Morse, Elizabeth A. Edwardsen, and Howard S. Gordon, "Missed Opportunities for Lung Cancer Communication," *Archives of Internal Medicine* 168, no. 17 (2008): 1853–58; H. M. Kim Marvel, Ronald M. Epstein, Kristine Flowers, and Howard B. Beckman, "Soliciting the Patient's Agenda: Have We Improved?" *Journal of the American Medical Association* 281 (1999): 283–87; Susan H. McDaniel, Howard B. Beckman, Diane S. Morse, David B. Seaburn, Jordan Silberman, and Ronald M. Epstein, "Physician Self-Disclosure in Primary Care Visits: 'Enough About You, What About Me?'" *Archives of Internal Medicine* 167 (2007): 1321–26; Dennis H. Novack, Neal A. Vaneslow, and Patricia A. Cuff, "The 2004 Institute of Medicine Report on Enhancing Behavioral Science Education: Can We Get There from Here?" *Annals of Behavioral Science and Medical Education* 11 (2005): 25–29; David B. Seaburn, Diane S. Morse, Susan H. McDaniel, Howard B. Beckman, Jordan Silberman, and Ronald M. Epstein, "Physician Responses to Ambiguous Patient Symptoms," *Journal of General Internal Medicine* 20 (2005): 525–30; Marc M. Triola, Henry Feldman, Adina L. Kalet, Sondra Zabar, Elizabeth K. Kachur, Colleen Gillespie, Marian A. Anderson, Cecily Griesser, and Mack Lipkin, "A Randomized Trial of Teaching Clinical Skills Using Virtual and Standardized Patients," *Journal of General Internal Medicine* 21 (2006): 424–29; Geoffrey C. Williams, Holly A. McGregor, Allan Zeldman, Zachary A. Freedman, and Edward L. Deci, "Testing a Self-Determination Theory Process Model for Promoting Glycemic Control Through Diabetes Self-Management," *Health Psychology* 23 (2004): 58–66.

5. Originally called the Task Force on the Medical Interview and Related Skills and then the American Academy on Physician and Patient, the AACH was an offshoot of the Society for Research and Education in Primary Care Internal Medicine (SREPCIM), an academic general internal medicine organization formed in 1978. Both the task force and SREP-

CIM grew exponentially, as general internists nationally assumed more medical student and residency teaching roles. Eventually, the task force (now the AACH) became independent of SREPCIM (now the Society of General Internal Medicine).

6. Sam Putnam graduated from Harvard Medical School and its Master in Public Health program. He spent two years studying in Ethiopia and then completed a residency in internal medicine in Seattle. He was director of a neighborhood health center in rural North Carolina and began research on the medical interview, which he called "interaction analyses." He continued this work after he returned to Rochester in 1984–88 to head the internal medicine residency at St. Mary's Hospital, an affiliated hospital of Rochester's medical school. During this time, Putnam participated in a two-month BPS fellowship with Rochester program graduate Mack Lipkin and also had interactions with Engel. After his untimely death in 2005, the AACH established the Putnam Scholars Program to honor his work.

7. Both are small groups led by trained facilitators, allowing providers to address countertransference issues that arise for them in the course of the medical encounter. The family-of-origin groups use a structured format, with each practitioner sharing his or her genogram. The personal awareness groups are somewhat more spontaneous.

8. Drossman and Novack, interviews.

9. Shimon Glick, a native of New Jersey, graduated from the SUNY Downstate College of Medicine. He trained in internal medicine at Yale University Medical Center and at Mount Sinai Hospital in New York City. In 1974 he immigrated to Israel and became chair of the Division of Medicine at the new medical school in Beer Sheva and later dean of the school and head of health services for the Negev region. His special interests have been in medical education, medical ethics, care of underserved populations, and palliative care. Under his guidance, medical school students experienced a curriculum that emphasized the social, geographic, and human dimensions of care (i.e., BPS medicine) and their special importance in primary care.

10. Shimon Glick, interview by Morse, April 2008; Sara Carmel and Shimon Glick, "Compassionate Physicians: Personality Traits and Prosocial Attitudes," *Psychological Reports* 73 (1993): 1362.

11. Dorith Shaham (director of the Patient Physician Communication Program for medical students at Hadassah Hospital, Hebrew University of Jerusalem School of Medicine), interview by Morse, October 2007.

12. Description of McMaster University MD Program, McMaster University Faculty of Health Sciences website, accessed March 12, 2012, fhs.mcmaster.ca/mdprog/social_community_context.html.

13. William Clark, e-mails to Morse, June 2007; Novack, interview. William D. Clark is a graduate of Harvard Medical School, an internist, past president of the AACH, and former medical director of the Addiction Resource Center in Bath, Maine. In addition to multiple activities with the AACH, he is managing editor of doc.com, a web-based comprehensive educational program in patient-physician communication and relationships, as well as psychosocial aspects of medical care.

14. Epstein et al., "Could This Be Something Serious?" 1731–39; McDaniel et al., "Physician Self-Disclosure," 1321–26; Seaburn et al., "Physician Responses," 525–30.

15. Typical of numerous comments students made to Jules Cohen in the 1980s and 1990s, when he was senior associate dean for medical education.

16. Moynihan, interview.

17. Epstein, interview.

18. Wendy Levinson, personal communication with Diane Morse, 1990. Levinson is professor and chair of medicine, University of Toronto, and former president of the Society of General Internal Medicine and the American Board of Internal Medicine.

Chapter Eight

1. Engel, "Need for a New Medical Model," 129–36.

2. Borrell-Carrio, Suchman, and Epstein, "The Biopsychosocial Model 25 Years Later," 576.

3. Herbert Weiner, "Is the Biopsychosocial Model a Helpful Construct?" *Psychotherapy, Psychosomatic Medicine, and Medical Psychology* 44 (1994): 73.

4. Borrell-Carrio, Suchman, and Epstein, "The Biopsychosocial Model 25 Years Later."

5. Edward Shorter, "The History of the Biopsychosocial Approach in Medicine: Before and After Engel," in *Biopsychosocial Medicine: An Integrated Approach to Understanding Illness*, ed. Peter White (Oxford: Oxford University Press, 2005), 9, 6, 10. See also Adolph Meyer, "Progress in Teaching Psychiatry," *Journal of the American Medical Association* 69 (1917): 861–62.

6. Graeme J. Taylor, "Mind-Body-Environment: George Engel's Psychoanalytic Approach to Psychosomatic Medicine," *Australian and New Zealand Journal of Psychiatry* 36 (2002): 449.

7. Lipkin, interview.

8. Bruce S. Singh, "George Engel: A Personal Reminiscence," *Australian and New Zealand Journal of Psychiatry* 36 (2002): 471.

9. Niall A. McLaren, "A Critical Review of the Biopsychosocial Model," *Australian and New Zealand Journal of Psychiatry* 32 (1998): 86–92.

10. Hamid R. Tavakoli, "A Closer Evaluation of Current Methods in Psychiatric Assessment: A Challenge for the Biopsychosocial Model," *Psychiatry* 6, no. 2 (2009): 25–30.

11. Richard Frankel, Timothy Quill, and Susan McDaniel, eds., *The Biopsychosocial Approach: Past, Present, Future* (Rochester, NY: University of Rochester Press, 2003).

12. Dennis H. Novack, "Realizing Engel's Vision: Psychosomatic Medicine and the Education of Physician-Healers," *Psychosomatic Medicine* 65 (2003): 929. Examples of this new research include Douglas A. Drossman, Yehuda Ringel, Brent A. Vogt, Jane Leserman, Weili Lin, J. Keith Smith, and William Whitehead, "Alterations of Brain Activity Associated with Resolution of Emotional Distress and Pain in a Case of Severe Irritable Bowel Syndrome," *Gastroenterology* 124 (2003): 754–61; Bing-Jiun Shen, Yael E. Avivi, John F. Todaro, Avron Spiro, Jean-Philippe Laurenceau, Kenneth D. Ward, and Raymond Niaura, "Anxiety Characteristics Independently and Prospectively Predict Myocardial Infarction in Men: The Unique Contribution of Anxiety Among Psychologic Factors," *Journal of the American College of Cardiology* 51, no. 2 (2008): 113–19; Andrew Steptoe, Katie O'Donnell, Ellena Badrick, Meena Kumari, and Michael Marmot, "Neuroendocrine and Inflammatory Factors Associated with Positive Affect in Healthy Men and Women," *American Journal of Epidemiology* 167 (2008): 96–102.

13. Novack, "Realizing Engel's Vision," 929.

Authors

DIANE S. MORSE, MD, is assistant professor of psychiatry and medicine at the University of Rochester School of Medicine and Dentistry. She is an internist whose present research and clinical activities—funded by the National Institute on Drug Abuse (NIDA 1K23DA031612-01A1), the McGowan Charitable Fund (Grant ID: 524475), and the Center for Medicare and Medicaid Innovation— focus on the application of self-determination theory to medical treatment utilization in criminal justice populations with psychiatric comorbidities. She has also published research on sequelae of family violence history, including childhood abuse and intimate partner violence, and on empathy and self-disclosure in patient-physician communication. Her activities during the period of this project were funded by the National Institute of Mental Health (NIMH T32 MH18911, PI Eric Caine, MD) and the Fulbright Scholar Program, United States Department of State.

KATHERINE R. JOHNSON, a freelance editor and writer, received a BA from the University of Pittsburgh, a BS from Kent State University, and an MS from the State University of New York at New Paltz. She has edited the *Official Bulletin* of the University of Rochester School of Medicine and Dentistry, articles on medical education, and the book *John Romano and George Engel: Their Lives and Work* by Jules Cohen and Stephanie Brown Clark.

JULES COHEN, MD, professor of medicine, attended the University of Rochester for both undergraduate and medical school. He interned at Beth Israel Hospital in Boston and returned to

Rochester for his residency and a year of postdoctoral training in hematology. He was then a research associate for two years at the NIH and a special research assistant at the Royal Postgraduate Medical School in London, England, where he received his training in cardiology. After thirteen years on the cardiology faculty at the University of Rochester Medical Center, he served for six years as chief of the medical service at Rochester General Hospital. In 1982 he became Rochester's senior associate dean for medical education and served in that capacity until 1997. As senior associate dean, he shepherded a major revision of the medical school curriculum and was administratively responsible (through others) for all medical student services and educational programs, as well as for the medical center's graduate medical education programs. During his years in cardiology, his research involved studies of cardiac hypertrophy, cardiomyopathy, and oxygen transport. In recent years, his work, research, and publications have been in medical education and in the development of a Health Professions Public Service Program, working with Karen C. Pryor (former associate dean for financial assistance). In 2000 he coauthored a seventy-five-year history of the URMC with former dean and vice president Dr. Robert Joynt. In 2003 he coauthored a biography of Dr. Paul Yu (former head of the Cardiology Unit) with Stephanie Brown Clark. And in 2010, again with Stephanie Brown Clark, he coauthored a historical biography of Drs. John Romano and George Engel.

Index

An italicized page number indicates a figure.

on depression, 21
on family medicine, 16–17
health care communication
    award for, 39
interviewing techniques of, 12
Medical-Psychiatric Liaison Unit
    of, 6, 19
photos of, *7, 22*
Reichsman and, 22, 23
research by, 16–17, 22, 24, 37
works by, 38
Epstein, Ronald M., 24, 26, 36, 43
health care communication
    award for, 39
at Highland Hospital, 25
photo of, *27*
research by, 27, 29–30
training of, 53n10
ethics, 14, 16, 39
ethnicity, as factor in disease, 37

family medicine, 16–17, 26, 35–36
Felten, David L., 34, 57n6
Ferris, Eugene, 2
Frankel, Richard, 25, 39, 55n22

gastric fistula studies, 16–17, 22
gastroenterology, 19–20, 37
General Clerkship, 6, 9
Genesee Hospital, 25, 26
geriatric psychiatry, 13
Glick, Shimon, 39–40, 60n9
Gold, Sandra, 31
Greene, William, 19, 20, 21, 45
Greenlaw, Jane, 14, 50n15
Guttmacher, Laurence, 8, 48n8

health care communication, 39
    interviewing techniques in, 12,
    38, 55n22, 59n5
    patient-physician, 29–30, 38, 39,
    41, 44, 61n13
Highland Hospital, 25, 26
HIV disease, 27, 37, 54n21
Hundert, Edward, 8

immune function, psychological
    influences on, 24, 33–34, 57n9
"integration conference," 9
Interpersonal Violence and Victim-
    ization Laboratory, 36
interviewing techniques, 12, 38,
    55n22, 59n5
Israeli Society of Medical Ethics, 39

Johnson, Katherine R., 63
Jozefowicz, Ralph, 12–13, 49n9

Kabat-Zinn, Jon, 49n5
Kaenel, Roland von, 38
Krasner, Michael, 12, 49n5
Kreipe, Richard, 56n5

Lambert, David, 29, 55n2
Lang, Valerie, 13, 50n10
Leading Organizations to Health,
    49n3
legal issues and ethics, 14, 16, 39
leukemia, 20
Levine, Maurice, 3
Levinson, Wendy, 39, 41, 61n18
Libman, Emmanuel, 1
Lipkin, Mack, 24, 25, 53n10
    on Engel, 45
    on patient-physician communi-
    cation, 37–39
lymphoma, 20
Lyness, Jeffrey, 13, 49n9

Markakis, Kathryn, 11, 25, 26, 48n3
McAnarney, Elizabeth, 56n5
McCann, William, 3, 19
McDaniel, Susan, 25, 36, 55n22
McMaster University, 40, 60n12
medical humanities courses, 13–15,
    14, 31
Medical-Psychiatric Liaison Unit,
    19–24, *20, 27, 33*
    establishment of, 6
    restructuring of, 24–27
Meyer, Adolph, 44